The Songs That
Saved Us

The Songs That Saved Us

My Dad, Dementia and Me

Simon McDermott

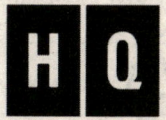

ONE PLACE. MANY STORIES

HQ
An imprint of HarperCollins*Publishers* Ltd
1 London Bridge Street
London SE1 9GF

www.harpercollins.co.uk

HarperCollins*Publishers*
Macken House, 39/40 Mayor Street Upper,
Dublin 1, D01 C9W8, Ireland

This edition 2025

1
First published in Great Britain by
HQ, an imprint of HarperCollins*Publishers* Ltd 2018

Simon McDermott asserts the moral right to be identified as the author of this work. A catalogue record for this book is available from the British Library.

ISBN: 978-0-00-871933-3

Printed and bound in the UK using 100% Renewable Electricity by CPI Group (UK) Ltd

For more information visit: www.harpercollins.co.uk/green

For my father

'You will go out in joy and be led forth in peace; the mountains and hills will burst into song before you, and all the trees of the field will clap their hands.'

Pride of Britain Awards,
November 2016

The lights were blinding.

I was sat surrounded by some of Britain's most famous faces – Simon Cowell, Stephen Hawking and Prince Charles. Two cameramen made their way over to my table, one positioning himself right in front of me. I could see the red light. I knew they were recording and my heart was pounding. On the stage, James Corden filled the screen, his voice booming across the room:

'There's a carpool karaoke superstar I want to pay tribute to this evening. He's 80 years old, he has the voice of Frank Sinatra and instead of Sunset Boulevard, he likes to cruise the mean streets of Blackburn, Lancashire. Ladies and gentlemen, I give you Mr Ted McDermott and his son Simon.'

The screen cut to a video of me driving with my dad in the car as he belted out 'Volare'. I felt pride and heartbreak all at once. There was the dad I knew and loved. He was happy and full of joy, with little sign of the confusion and aggression that had blighted our lives for the past four years. The interview cut to a picture of Mum and Dad when they were younger and then to Mum as she sat there with tears in her eyes: 'You do get upset about it. The person that you knew is slowly going away,' she said.

How did we get here?

My dad, Ted, was diagnosed with dementia in 2013, when he was 77. He can no longer recognize his family or where he is. It's been devastating to watch this insidious disease take him over, but through everything, music was the one thing that kept us together. Dad still loved to play his records at full blast as he sang around the house, remembering the words to every song, even though he didn't recognize anything else around him.

Living with dementia means that no day is ever the same. There were moments when Dad was happy and caring and moments when he would get incredibly angry and abusive but not know why. Some evenings he would often spend hours wandering around the house, shouting my mum's name, or looking for people who weren't there.

It was after one particularly bad outburst that I took Dad driving around the Ribble Valley in Lancashire, playing his old backing tracks to try and calm him down. It didn't take long before he was singing along in perfect tune. Dad – for a moment – was back to his old self and all the confusion and aggression had gone.

Those drives in the car gave us something to hold on to during the really bad times. I started to record them just for myself and Mum, but then I had the idea of uploading them to Facebook, with a link to a fundraising page I'd set up to support the Alzheimer's Society who'd supported us. In just a few short weeks the videos had been watched millions of times worldwide. The donations came pouring in and before I knew it we had raised over £150,000 for the charity to help other families like us.

Now I was about to go onstage to receive a Pride of Britain Award for raising dementia awareness. It was one of the most surreal moments of my life as Sir Cliff Richard and Dame Joan Collins appeared to present me with the award. 'I can't believe your dad sells more records than I do,' said Cliff.

For Dad, his one true passion has always been music. He's been singing since he was a young boy, growing up in a noisy house with thirteen brothers and sisters, and his musical ability was always encouraged. Although my grandparents didn't have a lot, the family never went short. My grandad was hard-working, with a job in the forge and lots of friends down at the local pub, while my grandmother was a strong and loving mother who knew everyone on the estate where she lived. Dad had a typical childhood for the time – his younger years were about football or playing out in the woods at the back of the estate. Once he left school, he worked in forges and factories but always sang on the side. Eventually, in his late thirties, he became a Butlin's Redcoat, where he travelled the country singing in clubs. He earned himself the nickname 'The Songaminute Man' because of the many different songs he could perform by heart.

Dad had just turned 65 when we started to notice his memory going. Mum picked up on it first – he would forget what he was doing, forget names and faces. Next came the frustration, the aggression and finally the realization that the person we knew was slowly fading away.

I'd always hoped Dad would write his own book one day – not least because he was a legendary storyteller when I was a kid. At family parties he'd often be found with a group of my cousins at his feet, enthralled by his stories. The tales would be greatly embellished, dramatic and over the top, but to young kids they were mesmerizing. One Christmas years ago, I bought him a blank notebook in which to write everything down, but dementia came and took away his past before he had a chance.

So it fell to me, his son, to capture as much as I could about Dad before he was lost to us for ever. This book documents his life growing up as the eldest of fourteen children in the Black Country, his life onstage, his loves, and then later the devastating effects of dementia on him and his family – as well as how he finally received the recognition for his singing that he always deserved. Things are very mixed up for

Dad – he can no longer tell his story without it becoming confused – so this is his story as told by others. I spoke to those people who knew him best: his remaining brothers and sisters, his friends, his teenage sweetheart and my mum, his wife of more than forty years. Where possible, these interviews have been used fully, alongside first-hand stories that Dad told me over the years. I've done my best to recreate them, though I know some stories will be for ever lost in time.

It was also important for me to include these stories so that Dad wasn't just remembered as a man with dementia who could sing. He was a singer first and foremost, who in later life was diagnosed with dementia. There is a difference. And to understand Dad's journey, it's essential to understand the man himself. His whole story matters – he is not his illness.

I so desperately miss my dad. Even though he's still around and I see him all the time, he's very much in his own world, and it's painful to watch Mum look after the man she loves. The thing is, when he was well I never really understood him for what he was. To me he was just Dad – the guy at home who would tell me off, get in the occasional mood, go out singing, love being the centre of attention, fly off the handle, care too much and be embarrassingly quirky. This book has become not only the story of my dad's life but my story, too. I've been given the gift of finally discovering the person my father is, why he behaves the way he does, his flaws, his weaknesses and his hidden strengths, which has, in turn, revealed to me who I am.

When I was young I thought my dad was the greatest man in the world. I lost that feeling for a while. But now I can say I'm the proudest man on the planet to have Ted McDermott as my father – the kind, the moody, the sensitive, the complicated, the brilliant, Songaminute Man.

This is his story.

My Kind of Town

Wednesbury is a small town right between Birmingham and Wolverhampton. It's part of the Black Country – so-called, according to Ted, by Queen Victoria in the 1800s. The story goes that Victoria was on a train being driven around the country when she looked out of the window to see the air thick with smoke from the many thousands of factories. 'This is such a black country,' she said, and the name stuck.

My father, Ted McDermott, was born in Wednesbury on 14 August 1936 to Hilda and Maurice McDermott. He was the first of fourteen children and a kind, cheeky, chatty kid who wasn't afraid to talk to anyone. His childhood was typical for a working-class family at the time. They weren't rich, but they had a strong sense of family and a determination to make the best of what they had.

Back in the Thirties, Wednesbury was a junction of goods yards, railways and factories. In the evening, the glow from the metal manufacturing lit up the sky for miles around. During the Industrial Revolution, hundreds of Irish settlers arrived in Wednesbury to do the digging – new roads, new railways, new everything.

The McDermotts were such settlers – the majority coming from Sligo on the west coast of Ireland. Legend has it that Dermot was one of the kings of Ireland before it was taken over by the English. Years later, Ted would sit and reimagine this history, telling his son that

Dermot was merely the poet to the King of Ireland. 'You're from a family of poets!' he would say.

It was against this industrial backdrop that Ted's parents were born and raised. Ted's mum, Hilda Carter, was born with warm red hair and a personality to match. His father, Maurice McDermott, was a quiet, small, thickset Black Country man who worked hard in the forge during the day, and would sing down the local pubs at the weekends whenever he could.

Like most young couples back then, Hilda and Maurice met locally and married quickly. Ted, their first child, was born soon after, followed with precise regularity by Maurice, Ernie, Fred and Colin. The young family were growing fast and in 1942 they all moved across town to the newly built 18 Kent Road in Friar Park – a council estate to the east of Wednesbury. It was the first time that a generation of McDermotts had moved away from Brickkiln Street, where Maurice had been brought up.

There was nothing lavish or luxurious about Maurice and Hilda's new house – it was small and red brick with a tiny garden at the front and a back kitchen leading out on to a simple back garden. It was spartan inside but the young couple soon made it their own, relying on hand-me-downs from family members and Hilda's thrifty eye. She could spot a good piece of material at 50 yards, barter over the price until it was within the weekly budget, and then manage to knock together two sets of curtains. No one had a clue how she could make so little stretch so far, but it was just as well given how many mouths there would eventually be to feed.

Hilda's shrewd money skills really came into their own during the war – while the McDermotts were entitled to more rationing coupons than most because of their swelling numbers, Hilda cut deals with the smaller, richer families, who would pay extra for the food the McDermotts got for less. Mrs Cook, who lived up the road and was a keen baker, would take Hilda's butter vouchers and happily give her back double the amount of margarine. Even without the food that was traded away, Hilda knew how to feed a growing family and would always have a pot on the go in the kitchen. She was friendly with all the local milkmen, bread men and grocers, doing deals with everyone and swapping her ration coupons like a pro.

The house changed very little over the years: there were three bedrooms upstairs – one master bedroom, a smaller back bedroom and a tiny single bedroom to the side. The toilet was out the back, to the side of the kitchen. The house might have been small, but it was their home and Hilda kept it as clean as she could. She was bright and entrepreneurial, and poured all of that skill into running a house and large family like clockwork.

It was the same routine every day, beginning with making sure Maurice had a proper breakfast to set him up for his day as a drop forger at the forge – a job he kept most of his life. Once he had gone to work, Hilda would turn her attention to the house and family. The kids were washed and fed, then she would prepare a pot of food for lunch and dinner, empty the fireplace of embers and re-lay it with sticks collected from the garden and coal pushed up the road in a wheelbarrow. Then followed the endless dusting, brushing bed-making and sewing, which Hilda tackled with her old apron tied around her waist and a cloth covering her hair.

Washdays meant boiling water on the gas stove before carrying it into the yard, where she washed and mangled sheets, clothes and nappies. Depending on the weather, these were hung out to dry either in the yard or in front of the fireplace, although they were always tidied away from view if Hilda had a visitor.

This was the backdrop to Ted's growing up.

A lot was expected of everyone and life wasn't comfortable compared to today's standards, especially when the other children – Mary, Jane,

John, Chris, Marilyn, Joyce, Malcolm, Gerry and Karen – eventually arrived. Hilda and Maurice slept in the tiny single bedroom at the back. The girls took the second smaller bedroom and the boys top-to-tailed in the larger master bedroom. Ted, being the eldest, had the single bed, while the rest of the boys slept in the two double beds. Each bedroom had a small window covered with Hilda's handmade curtains, and minimal furniture to make the most of the space. There were extra blankets for the really cold winter nights – not that they were often needed with everyone crammed side by side in the tiny rooms.

By modern standards, the house was cluttered – not in the sense that it was untidy or uncared for, but simply due to the number of young kids running about. The front door was always open, with Hilda's neighbours and friends either popping by to say hello or catch up on the local gossip.

Bedtime could often be chaos, with Hilda dealing with the girls first and then impatiently shouting the boys up to their room. Once everyone was in bed, she would close the door and the boys would be quiet until she went downstairs. The minute they heard the front-room door shut and knew the coast was clear, there would be a scramble for an extra jumper for warmth or a spare coat to use as a pillow.

It was often said that Ted was blessed with his father's caring nature, and growing up in such a tight-knit family meant that from an early age he developed a strong sense of responsibility towards them. Ted watched his father get ready for work every morning, and perhaps, on some level, the importance of providing for your family was impressed on him from a young age.

There were no holidays and very little spare money for treats, apart from on Sundays when Maurice would bring back a bag of sweets for all the kids. Although Ted's early years were hand-to-mouth, they were also spent finding fun outdoors. Come rain or shine, he and his friends would go looking for adventure right on their doorstep. Behind the house, outside the back garden, was Bluebell Wood. It had two ponds and was teeming with wildlife. Walking through the wood took you to old sewage beds, where the treated sewage was dumped and in the summer months methane would heat up the ground and steam pour out. Further on there were football pitches and 'The Jungle' – overgrown land full of silver birch trees. Ted, his siblings and friends from the estate would often play on this land in the summer, building dens, climbing trees and hiding out. It would be the first place that Hilda would look when calling the children in for their tea.

In those pre-television days, the young Ted was fascinated by nature. This was something encouraged by Hilda, particularly if he took some of his younger brothers and sisters outside with him to give her some peace and quiet. Ted could sense she had more than enough to worry about with the feeding and raising of so many children and, as a result, he soon developed a fantastic knack of knowing when to disappear. Hilda would often give the young Ted a spare slice of bread, telling him to go and sit in the garden and whistle for the birds to come. Sitting there, on the low stone wall, the birds would slowly but surely fly down out of the trees, pecking up the bread that Ted had scattered around him. He would sit there for hours if he could.

Life was bustling and busy, and there were plenty of local characters around to provide drama – one culprit being the local farmer, Mr Rumble, who owned Rumbles Farm. It was surrounded by cornfields, with small barns full of chickens and some pigs. Everyone was scared of Rumble – or Grumble as he became known – and all the local kids would dare each other to get anywhere near him. He didn't like children, especially those who trespassed on his land and would chase anyone away, no matter what their age, cursing and swearing as much as he could.

At the back of the farm ran Bescott railway marshalling yard. Hundreds of steam trains would park there overnight, and coal, which was being mined in the local pits, would be shipped around the country from the yard, while metals and goods that had been made at the factories nearby would be held in huge stores waiting to be transported. It was at the yard that all the big steam engines were repaired before they went back into service, and the railway line that passed through the town was the link connecting Wednesbury to the rest of the country – from Crewe further north to London down south. You could smell the oil before even setting foot in the yard – it was always in the air whatever time of year, but the scent was even stronger in the summer heat. All the carriage repairs took place at night and the tinkering of machinery and testing of engines could be heard long after the Friar Park residents had gone to bed. It became the reassuring sound that signalled bedtime for Ted and his brothers and sisters.

Maurice was close to all of his children, but he also worked long days, accepting all the work he was offered so that he could bring home as much extra cash as possible. It was Hilda who ran the household. Every Friday, Maurice would bring home a small brown envelope containing his wages and Hilda would take out what she needed to keep the house going, giving him back whatever was left for spending money. Maurice wasn't a big drinker, but he'd often let off steam down the local pubs, getting up and singing whenever he could.

Much of the manual work came from the two huge factories that were the epicentre of manufacturing around Friar Park – Elwell's and the Deritend. Elwell's made gardening tools and the Deritend Stamping Company was the forge where Maurice worked, which dated back to 1900. Its creation meant lots of jobs for men like Maurice, who lived locally, but there were also a number of people needing a wage who travelled in from across Wednesbury to work in such a steady environment. It was hard graft and long hours. Throughout the day, each time the hammers dropped, the boom could be heard right across Friar Park.

Every Christmas the factory held a party for all the kids and, when Ted was 5 years old, Hilda took him down to the club to join in the festivities. It was the first time he'd been to such a big party, and Hilda had sewn him a smart suit especially for the occasion. When they got there the room was full of young children running around; Christmas decorations brightened up the usually bleak, grey room and there were tables heaped with sandwiches, cakes and trifles. For Ted, this was heaven and he immediately found a small gang of kids to play with.

'Our Maurice will pick him up at five,' said Hilda to some of the women who'd organized the event.

'Behave yamself, Ted!' she shouted as she left the room.

The whole afternoon went brilliantly. It was something that Ted would remember all his life. There were party games like pass the parcel and musical chairs, a visit from Father Christmas, and enough sweets and trifle to sink a ship. At 5 p.m., just after clocking off from work, Maurice arrived to pick up Ted. The young boy was tired out, so Maurice carried him all the way home.

As soon as he got through the front door at Kent Road, Ted woke up. 'It was brilliant, Mom!' he said the minute his eyes opened, and he went on to excitedly talk about the afternoon he'd had, sparing no detail. Soon after tea, Ted was fast asleep again, so Hilda carried him upstairs, helped him out of his clothes and tucked him into bed. He was asleep the minute his head hit the pillow and Hilda carried his suit down to the kitchen, ready to wash it. She did the usual check of his pockets.

'What the hell is this?' she shouted. Her hands were full of jelly, cream and custard.

The suit was ruined. She was fuming.

'Have you seen this?' she shouted at Maurice, as if it was his fault. Maurice shook his head. He had no idea why Ted would do something so daft and he was angry that perfectly good material had been wasted.

The next morning Hilda was waiting in the kitchen when Ted came padding down the stairs, seemingly oblivious to what he'd done. 'You've ruined that suit, you have… shovin' all that food in there. Didn't you have enough to eat at the party?'

Ted looked distraught but Hilda suddenly realized what he'd done. 'I only brought the food home for the others, Mom, because they didn't get to come.' Hilda's heart melted. 'Yam bloody daft, you am,' she said and gave him a huge hug, explaining to him how he shouldn't put jelly and custard in his pockets again, no matter how much he wanted to bring it home to share with the others.

The McDermott household was a thrifty one and, like Hilda, Maurice was also resourceful. Sometimes, he and the other men from the estate would sneak through the fencing at the back of the house, make their way to Bescott railway marshalling yard and pick coal that had been delivered for the steam engines from the sidings. It was something that would be repeated every winter and, as the McDermott boys got older, more and more planning went into it. 'You could hear them all in the middle of the night,' says Ted's younger brother John. 'Us younger ones would all be tucked up in bed and then you could hear Ted, Dad, Maurice and a couple of their friends going through the fence at the end of the back garden.' Getting through the fencing was a mission, but once they were in, it was a free-for-all. 'It's what got us through those winters,' says John.

They were canny too: one day the lads became aware that there was a policeman down the road stopping locals suspected of taking the coal. So they decided to fill up some bags and hide them in the woods until the next morning when one of them could come back to collect them. It was a well-known fact that, if the copper did catch you, he would tell you off and confiscate the coal – before keeping it for himself.

'There also used to be a big tree at the end of the garden and, one winter, some of the blokes from the street all helped to saw it down,' says John. 'The whole street shared that wood for months.'

As they got older, Ted and his gang spent every minute together and as soon as he arrived home from school, he would be straight out the door playing with the other children in the street.

Often the boys would knock for each other and then go off the beaten track, mostly finding places where they shouldn't be. One day that involved heading far past the back of the woods, behind the football pitches, where there was an isolation hospital for people with infectious diseases. Patients with tuberculosis, smallpox and diphtheria were tended to by nuns; all the Wednesbury children were banned by their parents from getting too close. There were even rumours it was haunted. All the more reason to play knock and run… or so thought Ted. Although one day he wasn't quick enough and one of the nuns caught a glimpse of him as he knocked on the door and sprinted away. She marched to the house and told Hilda everything, meaning that Ted was rewarded with a smack from his mum and a warning of what would happen if he ever did anything like that again.

Smacks weren't rare: Maurice and Hilda were loving but strict. People sometimes assumed that children from big working-class families could get away with anything, but that wasn't the case with Ted's family. His parents were caring of course, but if any of the kids stepped out of line they'd come down on them like a ton of bricks. The kids knew that when they walked out of their front door they were representing the family, so they had to look smart and behave. Some mothers used to say, 'Wait till your dad gets home!' – but Hilda wasn't like that. She'd tell them off there and then and once they were disciplined, that was it; there was no waiting around until Maurice got home to give them a hiding. "Remember yow name!' Hilda used to tell the children. 'Because someone will come and tell me if yow do summat wrong.'

The first nine years of Ted's life were set against the threat, and then the reality, of war. When playing in the street, the young boys would often hear the distant roar of engines and, a few minutes later, they would look up and see the skies had turned black as the bombers flew across to Germany. Hilda and Maurice did all they could to keep things normal for the children, but the stark realities were impossible to hide and the constant threat of bombing was the main source of angst, even if the children enjoyed the drama. At the back of the house a small air-raid shelter had been built by Maurice just before the war started. Whenever the air-raid sirens went off, Hilda, Maurice and the elder McDermotts hushed the babies and placed them gently in drawers and covered them with blankets while the rest of the family squeezed into the shelter. As she always did, Hilda would stand on the doorstep shouting for all the kids by name, until every single one of them came running down the street and flying inside. Once they were all safely inside she would get in herself, satisfied that everyone was accounted for.

But life wasn't always dramatic and, even if the war did bring stress for the adults, the McDermott household was still one of routine, where everyone was expected to pull their weight. All the children had a job to do and they knew that they needed to get it done before playing out. Whether it was helping out Hilda in the kitchen, cleaning the carpets, folding the washing, clearing the garden or doing errands, everyone mucked in and did their part. Maurice would join in too at weekends, distracting himself and the others by breaking into song, giving them rendition after rendition of old classics as they mopped, dusted, changed bedding and beat rugs.

When time and money permitted, though, Hilda would treat the young Ted to a trip across town to Wednesbury Theatre to watch a variety show or musical. The performances were a typical mix of wartime entertainment – a defiance that the country's spirit would not be broken. The lights, the laughter and the sing-along songs were a refuge for them both. But to Ted, it was his first glimpse into a different world – a world of singing and sound – and a learning that, even in the hardest of times, the show must go on.

The eventual arrival of VE Day saw the whole of Friar Park out in the streets in celebration. Ted and the rest of the gang stood in the street as all the adults from the entire neighbourhood brought tables and chairs out for a huge party. Cakes were baked, bonfires were lit and drinks were poured. Ted had never seen anything like it in his life. The atmosphere was electric.

Normal life slowly resumed after 1945 and, to the children for whom air-raids and shelters were the norm, the war and all that came with it suddenly went away. The soldiers returned, the stories became fewer and the old rhythm of life returned to Wednesbury.

Baby Face

The veil of war eventually lifted and, although Ted was only young, the feeling of uncertainty the war had brought with it had a very real effect on him as it did on many others. To Ted, everything was temporary, and it soon became apparent that he had to enjoy every single day. He started looking for signs of life beyond messing about in the woods with his mates. While Hilda and Maurice carried on with the normal day-to-day routine, a curiosity opened up in Ted and, somehow, more seemed possible. But despite his dreams for something more, supporting his family was always the priority.

In his early teens, Ted took on as many odd jobs as he could handle, bringing in the extra pennies to help feed the still-growing family. He'd wake up at the crack of dawn to help deliver milk from the horse and cart, while every Monday he'd be wheeling an old pram around to all the women on the estate, collecting their husbands' suits and taking them to a pawn shop in Darlaston. On Friday he would pick them up again so all the men could be suited and booted at the weekend. Soon everyone around Friar Park knew Ted.

Around this time, Ted formed what would become a lifelong habit of trying out different things he thought would make him happy, with varying degrees of success. Like most other boys on the estate, he had a strong interest in football, but it was his love of music that was his true passion.

This musical love affair began with Maurice taking the teenage Ted along to the local pub, The Coronation – nicknamed The Cora – one Saturday night. The Cora was a huge pub, built in the early 1930s when the rest of the Friar Park estate was still under construction. Back then in the 1950s it was packed every night – it had a smoke room, a kids' room and a huge assembly room where bands could play. It was rough and ready but a magnet for local musicians and became known as *the* place to be. There he saw first-hand the magic of stepping up in front of the crowd and performing. Maurice would arrive like royalty, spend a few minutes chatting to his friends, and then be the first one up to sing. His favourite song was 'Marta' by Arthur Tracy and it was a real crowd-pleaser. By the end of his performance, the entire pub would be on its feet applauding. Maurice would then return to the bar, greeted by a series of backslaps and handshakes, before finding drinks lined up waiting for him as a young Ted looked on in awe.

Ted soon found himself walking in his father's footsteps when, aged 15, he left school and began working alongside Maurice at the Deritend forge. Everyone in the family had traditional roles – men went out to graft and Hilda would prepare a big, hearty lunch. It was sometimes Marilyn's (one of Ted's younger sisters) job to deliver it to the working boys, whose stomachs were groaning by midday. Everyone knew her down at the factory and would let her walk straight in – there was no Health and Safety in those days. As she watched them eat she was bowled over by how hard the men had to work, with the sweat pouring off them from their morning shift. 'All the men had sweated so much that, by the end of the shift, they could stand their trousers up because of all the salt,' she would say, years later.

The family work ethic was ingrained in Ted and he worked as much as he could, finally feeling he was earning his keep as well as bringing home a bit extra that he could spend on himself. He'd often work a 6 a.m. to 2 p.m. shift, come back home to Kent Road, then if there was extra work going, he would return to the factory and do the late shift until 10 p.m. At the end of the week he'd come home with his wages in a small brown envelope and hand it to Hilda, just like Maurice did.

'Come on, Big 'Un, yam a young lad, yam needing the money!' she'd say.

But Ted would have none of it: 'No, Muv, you need it more than me. Yam the one with all the mouths to feed! Buy one of the kids some new shoes. Our Jane could do wi' a new pair,' he'd say, walking out the kitchen before she could say anything else.

It was around this time that Ted and his friends began to head down to the local church youth club, nicknamed The Shack. It was free entry most nights, but on special occasions, when the organizer, Mr Turner, had booked a band or a singer, there was a small charge on the door. Those nights were like a military operation for Ted. He would pay a shilling to enter, then go to the toilets to pass his ticket to his brother Ernie, who would do the same to Maurice and Fred as they crouched outside underneath the window, hands stretched out to receive the illegal ticket.

On Saturday nights everyone made an effort to look the part, as it was the social highlight of the week for most of them – Ted's brother-in-law, Tony, remembers:

'All the boys wore their best suits and had their hair flattened down with Brylcreem. But however smart the crowd looked, it was Ted who always stood out. He'd walk in and command instant attention in his cream-coloured raincoat and white silk scarf. All the girls, whatever their ages, would swoon. He was the nearest thing to Dickie Valentine they'd ever seen.' Even then Ted had the women in the palm of his hand without really knowing it; he just had a presence that made everyone stop and take notice.

By now, Ted had stopped relying on Hilda's make-do-and-mend

policy when it came to his clothes. As he was growing up, Hilda had prided herself on making most of the children's clothes herself, going down to Birmingham Rag Market, buying second-hand garments, washing them, unpicking them, then sewing them all back together so they always looked brand new. But for Ted, that all stopped when he began to take charge of what he wanted to wear and carved out his own sense of style. He'd inherited Hilda's pragmatic approach to work and knew it was an important means to an end. If you wanted something, you had to look the part – that was half the battle.

That applied to making the right impression at The Shack. It was a small place with plastic chairs and tables, nothing fancy or glamorous, but it was always full. There was music and dancing, but Ted and his friends were there for one reason only – and that was to chat up girls. There was a routine to every Saturday night, which started with trolleys of tea and buns being brought round. Then the lights were turned down, the glitter ball switched on and the dancing began. Ted's brother Ernie was always the first on the dance floor and soon both brothers became popular with the girls – Ted because of his looks and Ernie because of his moves.

But it wasn't just Ted's dress sense that made him stand out. As soon as Mr Turner brought out the record player, Ted would be singing along. Like his father he appeared to have little fear of getting up onstage. After a while Ted became known for having a voice like velvet and the young audience couldn't get enough of him. They shouted and clapped and all sang along approvingly as he got into full swing. Being onstage, singing and entertaining a crowd was one of the best feelings he'd ever experienced and he soon became addicted.

One Saturday, after Ted and his friends had become regulars at the club, Mr Turner announced that they'd booked a professional singer for the following week, meaning that it was going to cost everyone an extra sixpence to get in. There was a lot of talk about who'd be coming. It was a big deal and everyone was wondering who it could be. The next week, the crowd was full of teenagers all dressed up in their best outfits, waiting to hear the mystery performer.

Eventually the singer arrived, dressed up to the nines in a tuxedo – you could have heard a pin drop as he handed his pianist the music. Then he started singing. It took the teenage crowd, who were used to Dickie Valentine and Jimmy Young, a while to register what was happening – there were no romantic crooning or show-stopping tunes; it was straight-down-the-line opera and it went down like a lead balloon.

'What the bloody hell is this?' a voice bellowed from the crowd and suddenly everyone else joined in, making it clear this was not the night they had expected. After his third song, the singer announced he needed a rest and would be back after a break.

'Dow bother!' someone shouted from the crowd. 'We dow want you back!'

By this time the whole room was booing and a near-riot was brewing. Mr Turner was trying his best to calm everything down, when suddenly someone shouted out: 'Ted! Give us a song!' Soon the whole crowd was chanting: 'Teddy Mac! Teddy Mac! Teddy Mac!'

The opera singer walked off the stage in disgust.

'And tek that pianist wi' ya!' shouted one of the boys.

Everyone jeered.

The pianist and the opera singer stormed out, with Mr Turner running after them apologizing. There was a huge cheer as Ted took to the stage and started to sing. He was up there for over an hour and he felt as if he was on top of the world, watching the crowd going wild, cheering him on and singing along. Ted had saved the day but, more importantly, in that moment he realized that this was exactly what he wanted to do with his life.

This moment of fame meant that Ted became a Saturday-night

regular, and he was soon packing out the club whenever he got up and sang. But it didn't take his brothers and friends long to work out that part of his attachment to the club was because someone had caught his eye – and they weren't wrong. Ted was bowled over the minute he spotted a girl named Iris across the crowded room. Iris was beautiful and stylish with thick, dark brown hair, and Ted soon forgot about the group he had arrived with. He plucked up the courage to go over and introduce himself.

At 17 years old there was no doubt that Ted was a charmer (Hilda always used to say that he'd definitely inherited Maurice's gift of the gab). He held out his hand and asked Iris for a dance. From that moment on, Ted began to court Iris with a winning mixture of innocence and determination.

Things settled into a romantic pattern quite quickly – they would meet at the club, dance and laugh and then Ted would walk Iris home and wait until she got safely into her house. After a few weeks of the same routine they had slipped into officially being a couple without anyone noticing – except for Hilda, who noticed everything.

There was no denying the mutual feelings – Ted was attentive, gentle and caring, making sure that Iris knew he liked her. Despite not having much money, he always saw to it that he gave her a little gift at the end of each date, even if it was just a slab of chocolate that cost him a shilling.

It was around this time that *The Carroll Levis Discovery Show* turned up in Birmingham searching for new talent. Carroll Levis was a God-like figure in the entertainment industry during the Fifties, a talent scout, impresario and radio personality – he knew what it took to be a star and could spot that quality a mile away. Ted read in the paper that his talent show was touring the country looking for someone with 'it' and he was determined to try out, taking the morning off work to go along. He took the bus from Wednesbury into the centre of Birmingham and made his way to the auditions alone. Although just 17, he was far from worried about having to get up and sing. Out of everything in his life, he knew that was the one thing he was good at. Ted knocked them out by singing 'Sweet Sixteen' and got through to the next round, which was a recording of the radio programme in London. But sadly it was not to be. As Jane, his sister, adds: 'No one really knows the full story as it's lost in time. It could have changed his life if he went. Someone once said that it was because the contestants had to pay insurance to appear on the show – something our Ted couldn't afford – so he didn't end up going.'

For now, singing professionally remained a dream that he couldn't afford to pursue, in more ways than one.

Ted bringing in a wage (along with the eldest of his younger brothers) did take the pressure off Hilda and Maurice and it allowed the younger boys to enjoy their childhoods in a relaxed way – they all loved football and they played for the local team. They devoted themselves to football in the same way Ted was committed to his music; the big problem was that the older brothers only had one pair of football boots between them, which often led to a big showdown.

Hilda soon cottoned on to this – but rather than keeping them under lock and key so that everyone got a turn, she thought this could be a valuable lesson for the boys: 'If you make the effort and get up early then you'll reap the reward.' The only thing she was adamant about was that all of them made sure the boots were clean and ready for the next person to use.

While the younger lads were bickering over boots and who scored the most goals, Maurice loved working with his eldest son and felt a huge sense of pride watching him learn the ropes. But despite the happy routine they had, which included Hilda making them both a full breakfast in the morning and putting out their work clothes, they both knew that National Service was looming when Ted turned 18.

He was a man now but that didn't stop the whole family dreading his departure – in many ways he was a big part of the glue that held the household together and a great support to Hilda, who wondered what would happen when he was away.

In the meantime, Ted and Iris's innocent courtship continued. Ted would take Iris to the bandstand to listen to music and sit on the bus holding her hand, telling her how beautiful she was.

'Yam the air I breathe,' Ted would tell her constantly.

'Come on now, Ted, yam embarrassing me,' she'd reply.

Looking back at this time, Iris recalls: 'Ted was always open about his emotions and wasn't shy about saying what he felt. But I was young and I used to get embarrassed when he'd tell me stuff. It's like he wanted everyone to know how he felt. I'd sit there holding his hand on the bus and I'd be bright red. He was ever so gentle, honestly. He would always tell me, "Yam beautiful." Looking back now, it was nice if you think about it...'

Iris was soon round at 18 Kent Road nearly every night of the week, waiting for Ted to finish work. 'Everyone loved Iris and she quickly became part of the family. Mom loved her being there,' says Ted's brother John. 'She'd help out around the house whenever she could, even looking after the little ones. She was ace.'

Iris had a very different backstory to Ted's – her parents had died when she was young (her father of a brain tumour when she was a toddler followed by her mother from tuberculosis when Iris was 11) and she had ended up being adopted by her nan. Ted found this heartbreaking. Given how close he was to his own parents and how much he enjoyed coming from a big and loving family, meeting Iris opened up a deep sense of emotion in him. 'I think he used to feel so sorry for me because I hadn't got a mum and dad and had to live with my nan,' Iris says now.

Despite a few emotional differences, the young couple found

something in one another and quickly became inseparable. They both had a good set of friends, but Ted had never been one to go off drinking with the rest of his mates. 'Honestly, he could sit with me all night, talking away about what he'd done that day and what we could do at the weekend, and that's how he liked it,' says Iris.

They slotted easily into each other's worlds – her friends thought she had struck gold with an adoring, older boyfriend who showered her with attention, his friends thought she was a stunner. Iris even became the football girlfriend, going along every Saturday to cheer on Ted from the sidelines. She would arrive with a big bag of oranges bought from the local fruit and veg stall, ready to cut them up and hand them out to the whole team at half-time.

But National Service was just around the corner, and before any of them could really feel prepared, they were saying goodbye to Ted as he went off for sixteen weeks of training in Litchfield, leaving Hilda full of worry and Iris counting down the days until he would return. Not knowing what was ahead of him, Ted put on a brave face, shouted goodbye to Maurice, kissed Hilda farewell and made his way down Kent Road to begin a new chapter.

Five Foot Two, Eyes of Blue

'There's room for the case underneath your bed. Put it away and be ready for inspection in five minutes.'

Those were the orders barked at Ted as he walked through the gates of Whittington Barracks – his new home rising to greet him as he tried to keep pace with everyone else. Although there were lots of rules and regulations, it soon became apparent this set-up made some of Hilda's rules back home look relaxed. Ted kept silent, quietly surveying the situation as the sergeant major stood shouting orders around the yard.

Those first few days and nights were long and filled with thoughts of what would be going on back at home. It was a big adjustment for Ted. At home he was Hilda's favourite, but now he was just one of many lads trying to stand out for all the right reasons, although that was hard as any attention given down the ranks was rarely a positive thing. However, slowly but surely, Ted's charm began to work its magic, and he started to make a real name for himself as he put his best into everything he did.

Physically he was also one of the fittest – the football training he'd done as a lad with his brothers stood him in good stead for the cross-country circuits, where he repeatedly found himself first back and barely out of breath. Gradually he built up a reputation at the barracks that was identical to the one he had at home – reliable, fun, kind and a great entertainer. That he was a great entertainer became obvious one

Saturday night a few weeks after he had joined, when he was asked to sing in front of the officers and their wives at their Christmas party. As he got ready to face the crowd and put on his perfectly pressed suit, it was hard not to think back a few years to the night he accompanied Maurice to The Cora. There, Ted had watched his dad closely as he sang away and had the whole audience on their feet.

Tonight it was his turn and, as ever, the crowd seemed to love it.

Life soon took on a reassuring pattern – being away from his family and Iris was hard, but Ted was always the one to roll up his sleeves, and enjoyed the rigour that Army life brought. He was top of the athletics and cross-country teams and wouldn't hesitate to step into the boxing ring for a few rounds. His knack of chatting to everyone and anyone whenever he could, soon meant he made a few good friends at the barracks. His best pal was Freddy Hyde, one of the officers' chauffeurs. Both men instantly got on. They shared the same sense of humour and enjoyed seeing how far they could push the status quo, a trait that was to reveal itself in more detail as time went on. Ted landed himself a job in the kitchen, quickly realizing that it was the best place to be as it kept you at the heart of things, as well as giving you access to any leftovers.

He soon became a firm favourite with both the officers and their wives: whenever there was a do on in the mess, Ted was always invited to sing. But it was the weekends that he lived for – it was his chance to get back to Kent Road to see Iris and the family. The first visit was allowed after he'd been away for a month, as the officers felt it was important for all the lads to bond for a few weeks and get used to their new surroundings. As the day of his visit home approached, Ted felt nervous and excited all at the same time. It felt strange not to speak to his brothers and sisters every day – he missed his family more than he'd thought possible.

Back at number 18, the feeling was mutual. Initially it was strange for the younger children to be at home without Ted and they missed the fact he wasn't there (though they were pleased to have the extra bed to sleep in!). The excitement was palpable the first weekend he came home. They sat by the window all morning waiting to hear the sound of his boots on the path and as soon as he walked through the front door, the younger children jumped on him for hugs.

Once everyone settled and a pot of tea had been made, Ted opened up his bag to reveal a stockpile of treats: fruit, butter, cheese and tins of meat. The family couldn't believe their eyes. Hilda was horrified: 'Get that stuff back in case they catch you!' she shouted. But he just laughed and said: 'Ah Mom, they'll just throw it out.' Ever the opportunist, Ted could see first-hand how much waste there was in the kitchen. At the end of every shift perfectly good food was thrown out (seemingly for no apparent reason, as it all looked fine to him). As far as he was concerned it wasn't technically stealing if it was just going in the bin; in fact he was doing a good thing applying the 'waste not, want not' principle when food was scarce. And so began the weekly ritual of Ted bringing home all he could to help the household eat, something that seemed to have stuck from childhood.

Despite living the high life at the barracks during the week, Ted was religious about his trips home. Once he decided to surprise his brother John and his friends, who were all about 10 years old and camping in the wood at the back of the garden.

'It was pitch-black when we suddenly heard this sound. We had no idea what it was, but we were terrified. We heard it move about and then stop right in front of our tent. We didn't dare move. Eventually we all fell asleep but when we woke up in the morning and crept outside, there was our Ted, asleep in his Army overcoat, using his rucksack as a pillow. He'd come home and Dad had told him to pop outside and check up on us because we were scared, but he'd slept outside all night to make sure we were OK,' says John.

Maurice and Hilda had always drummed into Ted the importance of behaving well in public. It was something that Ted would pass on to the younger ones whenever he could. 'He was ever so smart,' John explains. 'He would always tell us the importance of dressing well, the importance of how you behaved when you were out. I remember I had a football trial and he spent ages showing me how to press my trousers before I had to go down to the ground. Honest, he was forever looking out for us. I could never see any wrong in him.'

Ted felt proud to be able to come home and treat the family to some of the finer things in life – he wanted to share everything about his Army experience with them. One day, Hilda was looking out the front window when a big posh car made its way slowly down Kent Road towards their house, eventually parking right outside. 'Oh, look at this!' she shouted to everyone. 'What's this big car doing outside our house?'

Hilda wondered who their visitor could be – that was until she saw a familiar grin as one of the car's windows slowly wound down. 'GOOD GOD! They'll get sent to bloody hell if they get caught,' she yelled. Maurice and the kids weren't quite sure what was going on. The next thing there was a knock on the front door and it was Ted and Freddy, dressed up in suits. They had arrived in the officers' shiny car, complete with all the flags flying on the front. The younger kids couldn't believe their eyes but Hilda went berserk as the two boys stood outside on the doorstep, laughing their heads off.

No matter the occasion, Ted always loved a good suit. A few weekends after his first homecoming, he showed up wearing a full tweed outfit, complete with shooting stick from one of the officers. Again, Hilda nearly had a fit when she saw him and screamed: 'Get that off! You'll be in the Jankers [Army prison]!'

But nothing seemed to faze Ted. Pretty much every weekend when the officers were away, he'd come home wearing their best clothes – a different outfit every week – and go out in them to the local clubs, enjoying feeling like a millionaire and having the time of his life. After a few months he even turned up in a full evening suit – black tie, white shirt, even the hat – a double of Dickie Valentine. The next day, everything would be washed, dried and ironed to perfection with none of the officers being any the wiser.

It became a regular thing, especially if Ted was taking Iris out on a Saturday night. Once Hilda got over the worry that Ted would end up in jail, she would get emotional every time she saw him all dressed up. Maurice was less sentimental. 'Teddy Bloody Big Head,' he'd say. 'Look at him, he acts like he owns the bloody street!' But secretly he was full of pride and would go down the pub, telling everyone how well his son was doing and that he was destined for great things.

Freddy Hyde became part of the family, and would be around Kent Road as often as he could. One day, he turned up to surprise Hilda: 'Come on, Mrs Mac, get in the car and I'll tek you for a ride up to Worcester.' Off they went, with Freddy chauffeuring Hilda for a day out, helping her pack the bags and then driving her the long way home so that they would be seen cruising through the Wednesbury streets in a smart car, imagining the twitching curtains. Ted would also impress Iris with the car when they went out. Saturday night was their time together and they would still go down to The Cora, where he had started to be greeted as a bit of hero, especially if he gave in to the persuasion of the crowd and took to the stage for a few songs. They were happy days, topped off only by the sense of pride the family felt as the day of Ted's passing-out parade arrived.

Hilda was bursting with joy at the fact that Ted had passed his training and was serving his country, so there was much excitement when they found out that the parade would pass through the centre of Wednesbury. All the younger children were full of anticipation, not least as their school would be closed in honour. When the big day arrived, the main street completely shut down and people gathered along both sides of the pavement – it was just like the end of the war all over again. Hilda put on her best dress and made sure all the kids were as smart as they could be, warning them all to be on their best behaviour and do their brother proud. Ted's brother John was there on the day: 'All of us went down to see Ted, including Iris. Mom made sure we were in prime position. All of a sudden we could hear the brass band. It was getting louder and louder as they came down Lower High Street. I was trembling with excitement.'

As the soldiers approached, Hilda kept shouting for everyone to look out for Ted. John spotted him first. 'Mom! Mom! Here's Ted!' he shouted. Suddenly, he was right there in front of them and the whole family was shouting 'Ted! Ted! Ted!' and cheering him on. As he passed, he gave them a wink and a smile and then he was gone – it was all over in a flash. John turned to speak to their mother and saw her wiping away a few tears.

'Why yam crying, Mom?' he asked.

'I'm not crying, I'm happy,' she said. 'His Dad would be so proud.'

Ted was feeling elated. Hearing Hilda, Iris and his younger siblings all shouting his name gave him the same buzz he felt when he got up onstage.

Afterwards there was a big do at the officers' mess with food and drink and families mingling. Ted introduced Iris to the rest of his mates and everyone stood around making small talk. After a little while one of the officers started talking to Hilda and eventually ushered her through into a separate room. She was greeted by an officer she hadn't met before.

'Mrs McDermott, how do you do?'

'Very well, thank you,' said Hilda, smiling.

'I wanted to say what an absolute credit your Ted is to you, one of the team and what a cracking singer, that voice!'

They both stood there making small talk, but Hilda could sense that he was leading up to something. Deep inside her she knew what it would be and she dreaded it.

She asked him outright: 'Yam sending him abroad?'

'We might be,' he said.

Hilda paused, aware of who she was talking to, and finally replied: 'I hope you don't. He's got thirteen brothers and sisters and I rely on him.'

'I'll see what I can do,' he said.

So that's how Ted didn't get posted abroad when he was in the Army. Instead he became a batman – a soldier assigned to a commissioned officer – and his chores involved cleaning, serving food at mealtimes and sorting his clothes as well as doing any errands. In effect, he managed to have a role that was important but which involved none of the danger.

It seemed a bit of a charmed Army experience and a world away from some of the hardships suffered by others. Ted's brother-in-law Tony was there at the same time: 'Every time we'd be training, he'd be walking around the camp like he owned the place. We'd be training hard and covered in sweat and he'd just wander off out the gate. I don't know how he bloody got away with it.' Ted even found a way to leave camp every night and cycle across town to see Iris! His obsession with being meticulous about his appearance and well turned out was reinforced by his new role – his shoes always had an extra shine and he was never ready for the day unless he was wearing a tie and a sharply ironed suit.

The way Ted had managed to include the thing he still loved the most – music – in his work life was also a brilliant stroke of luck. As the months went on, his confidence and reputation grew and so did Iris's pride in her boyfriend's talent. Things between them were going well. They were officially 'steady' and would often spend evenings out with Hilda and Maurice. During Ted's weekends off, the four of them would make their way to The Cora.

From 7 p.m. every Saturday, people would have to queue to get through the doors. Most weeks there was a skiffle group playing – a group of local musicians (realistically this meant anyone who could play a homemade instrument) that featured Desi Mansel on the drums, Ted's younger brother Ernie on the bass (which was actually a tea chest with lengths of string tied to it), and anyone who could play the piano. A guy called Teddy Price also sang. He was cross-eyed with big ears and buck teeth and whenever he began to sing he'd shout out to the females in the crowd: 'Look at the eyes, girls, look at the eyes.' Another singer there was Kenny Kendrick, who lived next door but two to the McDermotts. He fancied himself as a bit of an Al Jolson, and always carried a pair of white gloves in his pocket in case he needed to sing. These nights stood out for Iris, who adored being part of such a large and loving family: 'We all used to get dressed up, me, Ted, his mum and dad, and make our way down to The Cora. Ted was always dressed immaculately. Those nights were some of my best memories from when I was younger. It was packed. Maurice would always be the first one to get up and sing – he had a wonderful voice – he'd always sing, "You're Nobody 'Til Somebody Loves You". Ted started singing that song, too. Later on in our relationship, he used to say to me, "If I can't see you, look at the clock at 11 o'clock and I'll be singing, 'You're Nobody 'Til Somebody Loves You'". And I'd have to play that record then.'

It was Iris who first realized that there was more than a hint of anxiety behind the apparently confident Ted just before he stepped onto the stage. The stress would come on just as he was gearing up for his turn in the spotlight, and he would suddenly start rubbing his nose. It became a telltale sign that the nerves and excitement were threatening to overwhelm him. Iris understood that it was less about being shy (after all, Ted could easily step up onto the stage in front of total strangers) and more like an energy that he couldn't control. And once she started noticing this anxiousness before Ted's performances, and as she got to know him better, it soon became clear that offstage he could easily become downbeat and gloomy without a performance to look forward to.

Ted worked hard to keep these feelings to himself, especially as it really wasn't the done thing for men to discuss such things in the 1950s. He also knew, once he left the Army and began working, those feelings couldn't make an appearance. Deep down Iris knew that he needed love, affection and reassurance to keep him on an even keel and she worried about him, but nevertheless they had a volatile relationship and he sometimes had mood swings that tried her patience.

Eventually, after three years together and despite the rows, Ted decided that he wanted to make Iris his wife. Perhaps he thought it would help bring a much-needed calm to their relationship. Ever the romantic, he planned his proposal meticulously and to add to the sense of occasion, he decided to do it around Christmas 1956. Hilda was delighted that her eldest son was settling down – she liked Iris being around and she was practically part of the family anyway. But having a ring on her finger didn't necessarily put an end to their problems or Iris's concerns: 'That ring was in the garden more times that it was on my hand,' she laughs. 'He would get very jealous. I think two weeks after he gave me the ring he told me he wanted it back! His friends used to come up to me and say, "Oh, you look nice, Iris," because they knew it would wind him up. I'd tell him not to be silly but he would sulk afterwards like I'd been flirting with them!'

Iris and Ted did get engaged and stayed that way for years – certainly more than most couples who had decided to spend the rest of their lives together, but they finally split up in the early 1960s when Ted was 24 years old. All these years later, even Iris isn't really sure why their great love affair came to be over.

'Why did it end? Oh, I don't know. We had one of our usual arguments – he was very possessive of me and always worried I'd go off with another bloke. But this argument was just a lot bigger and it lasted a lot longer than the rest and we never got back together,' she says. 'I started seeing my husband soon after. Ted disappeared and my husband came along – nice car, wonderful job – he had everything and I was married to him twelve months later. I had grown up with nothing and I wanted to have a different life.'

Ted's version of the break-up was very different and, as Iris says, steeped in his fear of Iris leaving him for another man. According to Ted, both of them were holding down two jobs – Ted had left the Army by then and gone back to working double shifts at the Deritend from six in the morning to ten at night, while Iris was working at Elwell's during the day and at the Hippodrome cinema in the evening. One day Ted came home from work early and Hilda asked him if he was OK. Ted told her that he didn't feel right and so had finished work early. Hilda cooked him something to eat, he had a bath and then he decided to go into Wednesbury to see Iris. He drove down on his bright pink scooter – a DKR Dove – and waited outside her work to surprise her. But instead, according to Ted, he watched Iris come out of the cinema and get on the back of the motorbike belonging to one of Ted's friends in the Army. They had words and the engagement ring went over a garden wall at the bottom of Rydding Lane. Ted didn't tell anyone and went straight to bed as soon as he got home.

The next day, Hilda got up to make breakfast and start the daily chores. She went straight to the boys' bedroom and pulled open the handmade curtains, where she found Ted still in bed. She had no idea why he hadn't gone to work and was just about to start quizzing him, despite the fact he was pretending to be asleep, when suddenly there was a loud bang coming from the front of the house as the gate slammed shut and someone started hammering on the front door. Hilda peered through the curtains in the front bedroom and saw that it was Iris's nan making all the noise. She went down to calmly open the door and started to speak, but didn't get a chance to say a word before the woman launched at her:

'I wanna see your Teddy. I wanna know what he's said to our Iris. Hers crying her eyes out and she won't go to work.'

Hilda still had no idea what was going on and shouted upstairs for Ted to come down and explain himself. Ted came down the stairs in just his trousers, slipped his bare feet into his shoes, calmly put on his jacket and walked past the two women stood on the step. 'I dow wanna talk about it. I'm going,' he said.

That was the last time Hilda and the family saw Ted for over three weeks. Everyone was distraught and worried – even Iris who told Hilda she hadn't seen him but didn't give the whole story about the row and the concerns she'd had before they split up. Then one Sunday dinnertime, Ted's nan came over and told Hilda that he was safe with her. The whole road must have heard Hilda exhale with relief. 'He's alright – just give him some time,' she said. However, Ted hadn't left the house once since arriving at his nan's.

The next day Hilda went over to Walsall to try and persuade Ted to come home, but as soon as he saw her coming up the path, he walked out the back of the house, too embarrassed to be seen like that by his mum.

Eventually, after a number of failed attempts, Hilda finally managed to persuade him to come home. She warned everyone back at Kent Road not to say a word about Iris to Ted and on the night of his return, while the rest of the family were sat in the front room, Ted opened the front door, went straight upstairs to bed and didn't speak to anyone. He stayed in his room for days. It was a low point for the whole house to see Ted in that state. His sister Jane says: 'After a while he got over it, though – and that's when he really started to enjoy his life.'

But no one really knew until years later how deeply the end of the relationship had affected Ted.

Consider Yourself

On the face of it at least, things soon went back to normal for Ted. His National Service had ended after a lively eighteen months, and everyone was relieved to see him getting on with things. But what they didn't glimpse lurking beneath the happy-go-lucky demeanour was discontent: Iris's observations about Ted's tendency to feel anxious were well founded. To Ted, everyone else seemed to have their lives sorted – jobs, partners and children, a clear life plan, but his structure had fallen away. He didn't have the discipline of the Army, or a house or a car or anything really; all he owned were his records. Ted wasn't so much driven by making money or having material goods, despite his love for a quality suit and looking the part. Instead, his enjoyment in life came purely from making people happy – from entertaining and putting on a show.

The late 1950s and early 1960s were a relatively prosperous time across the country, but nevertheless making ends meet was hard for a lot of families. Ted still witnessed Maurice and Hilda watching every penny and he continued to make sure that any extra he had went into the household. Leaving the Army had been a blow for him, and returning to the factory, seeing all the old faces still there, plugging away to make ends meet, felt like taking a step backwards. His brothers and sisters were growing up and one by one leaving the family home. Life slipped back into a familiar pattern: the only thing missing was having Iris as his girlfriend.

That said, it was impossible for Ted to fully close the door on that relationship, mainly as Iris would still come round the house to see Hilda. The two women had formed a strong bond and neither was ready to cut the other off completely, despite the break-up. Ted tried to take this in his stride and was relieved that these visits would often take place before he finished work. However, there was the odd occasion when Iris's perfectly timed exit didn't quite pan out. It all came to a head about a year or so after the couple had split up and Ted came in from work to find Iris still there. He went into the kitchen to put the kettle on, as he did every night he came home, and handed everyone a mug of steaming tea, everyone except Iris.

'Where's mine?' she asked.

'In the kettle. You can make your own,' he replied.

The hurt between Ted and Iris still ran deep in him, so he clutched on to a new daily routine to bring him order and structure. He wasn't remotely interested in finding a new girlfriend and instead started spending time with his brothers – down at the club and out and about. His brother John remembers: 'After he came out of the Army, Ted would spend hours polishing his shoes – so much so that you could see your face in them. If I was going somewhere with the school, he'd show me how to tie my tie. He'd say, "Come here, you. You ay going out like that. I'll show you how to do a tie," and he'd sit there and show me.'

Friday night was the real performance though – everything had to be perfect and even his handkerchief would be pressed and placed across the top of his jacket pocket in a neat line.

Before he went out, Ted would make sure that Hilda had given him the once-over: 'What do you think of this, Muv?'

'Looks alright, Ted,' she would reply.

Then he'd head back upstairs to finish getting ready. A few minutes later he'd be back in the kitchen with the handkerchief refolded in a different style – this time with three points to it.

'You think this one looks better?' he'd ask.

'Well, yeah, it's alright,' Hilda would say, not really paying attention.

This performance would usually repeat itself until Maurice looked up from his newspaper and bellowed: 'FOR CHRIST'S SAKES, it's a bloody handkerchief!' But in spite of this, he was delighted to see his son looking the part. He'd watch Ted walk out of the front door and up the path with quiet delight, often turning to his wife and saying: 'Look at him, our Hild. He walks down that street thinking he's a bloody millionaire! He might not have a penny in his pocket but he's singing and whistling to himself like he hasn't got a care in the world.'

Being well turned out became one of Ted's defining features. But his quest for the perfect 'look' often meant that if he didn't have the outfit he wanted, he would simply borrow from his brothers in order to create the right style. His brother Colin was the usual target: 'I remember one time I'd just got paid and bought myself a new top from Burton's one Saturday. I'd come home, had my tea and then Ted goes, "Col, can you lend me half a quid?" I said, "I can, but yow gotta start looking after your money a bit better, our Big." Anyway, me and Micky Felton went up the Adelphi and then afterwards we popped into the Star and Garter for a drink. Who was sitting at the bloody bar? Our Ted, smoking a little cigar with half a Guinness… and wearing my bloody new top. I didn't say anything and asked him if he wanted a drink. The next day I asked our mum, "Did Big have my new top on last night?" "No," she'd say, and would always cover up for him. He could do no harm in her eyes!'

In fact, Hilda was happy to aid and abet when it came to Ted 'borrowing' his brother's clothes – if he wore one of Colin's suits the next day, she would brush it down and hang it on the line to air it out.

Despite having regular gigs at The Cora and the many other pubs in Wednesbury, Ted would hardly drink. 'You could buy him half a shandy and you'd be hard-pressed to see if it had gone down by half an inch by the end of the night,' says John. 'On the nights that he was singing, he'd have a glass of tea – everyone used to think that he'd be drinking neat whisky. That's what kept him so fit.'

Family loyalty was everything for the McDermotts, and Ted led the way in making sure they weren't disrespected. He had a bit of clout locally – a good job at the factory, a successful Army record and a great voice that dominated the local clubs. A few years after coming back from the Army, he continued this tradition while defending his niece, Lorraine. She was the daughter of his brother, Fred, and his wife, Edna. From a young age, Lorraine had suffered with a slow eye, which meant she had to wear a big patch over her glasses to correct it. One day she went to play at a friend's house – it was the Spooner family and they had lived on the same street as the McDermotts since Ted was a boy. All the children had grown up together, playing out and getting into all sorts of scrapes, and their parents went to The Cora together on a Friday night.

None of that mattered to Ted as soon as he saw Lorraine bolt through the front door in tears. 'What the bloody hell's happened?' he shouted. Lorraine didn't want to say anything at first but eventually he persuaded her to tell him – it turned out that one of the Spooners had said it would bring bad luck on the house if Lorraine looked directly at her with her bad eye. Ted didn't wait around to hear the rest of the conversation – he marched to their house and banged on the door with the force of a hurricane. As soon as Spooner opened the door to see what all the racket was about, Ted knocked him out with one clean punch. As he left Spooner out cold in the hallway, he shouted over his shoulder: 'Dow you talk about our kid like that again.'

A few weeks later, Ted and Spooner were down at The Cora again having a drink and listening to music, no grudges held but a point made and a warning thrown out to anyone else who tried to disrespect his family.

Ted couldn't stand to see anyone being treated unfairly or taken advantage of, regardless of the situation, and he'd often speak up or step in to defend anyone he felt was being mistreated. Ted wasn't scared of authority either, and if the people in charge were the ones upsetting anyone in the family, they got the same treatment. One day, when his little brother Malcolm was only about 12 or 13 years old, he came home from school sobbing and with food around his face, saying that the teacher had shoved his head into his dinner because he hadn't finished his vegetables. Ted saw red and went striding down the road to the school, to find this so-called teacher and see what he had to say for himself. As he turned the corner, he saw two policemen waiting and as he approached, they put out their hands to slow him down: 'Steady on, mate. We know why you're here but you need to calm down!' It turned out that as soon as the teacher realized the boy he'd attacked was a member of the McDermott family, he told the headmaster and decided to call the police in anticipation of trouble. It seemed that Ted's reputation for protecting his own went before him.

It wasn't often that the kids went home and confessed to being in trouble with a teacher, as they knew they would get an extra clip round the ear for being a pain at school. But something like this was different, especially with a family that didn't take too kindly to any sort of disrespect. The teacher couldn't apologize quickly enough to Ted, who simply replied: 'It's not me ya gotta apologize to, it's me brother you need to say sorry to.' Once the matter was sorted, the second policeman took him aside and said: 'If I were you, mate, I'd wait for him and I'd give it him. If that was my brother, I'd make sure he wouldn't do it again.' But Ted felt he had dealt with the situation – his sister Chris avows: 'Our Ted wasn't violent, he wasn't like that at all, but he would always stick up for what was right. If anybody said anything, well, that was it. He wouldn't let anyone put on we.'

★★★

In his early twenties, Ted was well known around the pubs in Friar Park for getting up and singing whenever he could. But despite working in the forge during the day, it was a chance meeting with an old Army mate, Tommy, that took his life in a different direction.

They were catching up over a drink one night, putting the world to rights, when Ted was offered an opportunity he couldn't turn down. Tommy's dad worked at Walsall Football Club and had told him about the need for an announcer at the matches. Ted grabbed the opportunity with both hands – not only would it give him the extra pennies for his pocket, but it would also allow him free entry to the match as well as being able to put his vocal talents to good use.

After a quick training on how to use the Tannoy system, he soon had a regular gig every match day down at the club. As well as the standard announcements, he would entertain the crowd by playing records and reading out the raffle results. He was in his element. He slowly made a name for himself with the managers at the club, mainly as he wasn't afraid to speak his mind, sharing ideas about what he thought would help contribute to the club's success.

'You gotta bring the women in more,' he told one of the directors. 'Get them in and the blokes will follow.'

It was a good idea. Soon the club was putting on a 'posh' buffet with drinks after the match. Music was the perfect accompaniment – which gave Ted the opportunity to perform alongside some big and brilliant acts. The platform was way more substantial than at the local clubs, the crowds were bigger and the nerves more palpable, but the adrenaline rush was just the same. The success of the events meant that Ted was given a full-time job at the club and put in charge of promotions, enabling him to leave the forge.

It was also a dream come true for Ted's brother John. He was football-obsessed and took Ted's job as an opportunity to be down at the club whenever he could. Ted had been there a few months when he came home one night shouting for John to 'Get yer boots on! We'm a player short at Walsall and we need you to come down and play for a second team.' John couldn't get down there quick enough and played a blinding match – he wowed them all so much that they wanted to sign him up there and then. But doing so would have meant walking away from a steady job just when he was about to get married, and he had to pay the bills, not 'run around a pitch for a living and hope it would fill the electricity meter'. These were obviously the days before players could earn a fortune and John became one of a long line of McDermott men who had to push aside their dreams for the sake of providing a roof over the heads of their loved ones.

Because the McDermott boys did pull their weight, they were never out of work despite the turbulent times, and Hilda felt proud to have raised them. As they got older, the priority was no longer pulling them out of bed for school, it was setting them all up with a good breakfast and clean clothes for a heavy day at work. One by one that responsibility became another woman's, as each of the sons married and moved out.

Ernie, Maurice and Fred tried to make their money away from the factory; the three of them worked at a huge slaughterhouse, killing over 1,000 pigs a week. Ernie inherited Ted's knack for spotting a way to bring home extras and always managed to snag a few slices of meat, making sure that his mum and the rest of the family had food. Like all families at the time who were trying to make ends meet, the McDermott boys loved to see how bold they could be when it came to sneaking extras. Each was full of charm and worked so hard that no one minded if they took some slices on the side. It was the same story in most workplaces, if the boys put in the hours, bosses were happy to turn a blind eye. There are many stories about how Ernie once came home after work with a row of sausages wrapped around his waist, tucked under his shirt away from sight. Eventually, his brother Maurice became one of the deliverymen – which meant even more meat for Kent Road. 'No one starved in our house,' he used to say. But Hilda also made sure her friends down Kent Road never went short. She would often cook big pots of stew and share them with the neighbours. Years later, Ted's sister Chris was walking to work when she bumped into her old friend Marilyn, who also grew up on Kent Road. She was there with her mother-in-law. 'This is Chrissy Mac,' Marilyn said. 'Do you remember me telling you? If it wasn't for that family, we would have all starved to death.'

The boss of the slaughterhouse, Mr Hollinsworth, was a fan of the McDermotts, often saying to Fred as he left on a Friday: 'Tek that for your dad's tea', and handing him a few slices of something for the weekend. Ernie and Maurice had other odd jobs, too – it was very much a family affair and they all did their bit to try and take some of the pressure off Maurice and Hilda whenever they could.

Although having a job for life would have provided some security, it just wasn't like that in Ted's part of the world in the late 1950s. You had to be nimble and willing to turn your hand to almost anything because things were changing all the time. So when work at the football club dried up, Ted had to weigh up the reality of working somewhere in town with fewer paying shifts just so that he could sing against moving on and taking more regular work with better pay. The need for a regular wage won the day and Ted, Fred, Maurice and Ernie all ended up getting jobs with Wimpey, a company who were building new homes around the Midlands in places such as the Woods Estate, Bulls Hill and Hollyhead Road.

Ted got a job as a watchman on one of these sites and immediately earned himself a reputation as a lovable joker, sticking his head in the cement mixer and singing a tune, asking them what it sounded like. He was always singing and, just as in his Army days, constantly dreaming of other things. He always made sure he did the job in hand and was respectful to his co-workers and bosses, but he found it hard to concentrate on anything that wasn't music, so the job was a godsend.

Ted's wheeling and dealing became legendary – especially when he went through the phase of offering to put on bets for some of the blokes on the building site. He and his mate Georgie had more freedom than the rest to come and go from the site and were able to slip away to place bets for all the workers, who were almost religious about gambling. One day a chap gave them a double bet to put on. Ted was adamant he had backed the wrong horse and wouldn't win, and so he and Georgie decided to keep the money instead.

Ray Barns worked on the site with Ted and knew that he hadn't placed the bet and so was keeping an eye on the race for him – the next thing you know he's bursting through the doors to where Ted was quietly having a cup of tea on his break and shouting: 'Ted, Ted! That horse has only gone and bloody won 100 to 8!' They all dashed back to the betting office, praying the chosen horse wouldn't win the next race. It was neck and neck and went to a photo finish. Ted and Georgie were panicking because they were about to lose a month's wages each. Luckily for them the horse lost; it was probably one of the closest calls he had.

Moving forward, Ted's varied career included working for the council in the gardens, often driving home for his lunch in a dumper truck he'd 'borrowed' (despite not having a driving licence), and then working for the water board. He wasn't beyond enlisting the younger kids to earn extra cash either, telling them to keep their eyes peeled for a leak in the street, as he would get paid extra for spotting any and reporting them.

Weekends were still a time for Ted to let down his hair and now that he was that bit older and had more spare cash, he would travel further afield than The Cora. He started popping up to Taffy Griffiths Coach Station on Crankhall Lane in Wednesbury. He'd chat to the coach drivers to find out where they were headed and if he fancied it – usually Blackpool or Worcester – would ask if they had a seat and off he'd go. He didn't have a grand plan and was happy to travel where the wind took him. Not shy of talking to strangers and in search of a new adventure, he would pal up with someone on the coach and end up singing in an unknown bar or club, where they'd often have a collection for him, before heading back on the first coach the next morning. After a while most of the drivers got to know him and would let him sleep in the back of the coaches – sometimes they'd even wait for him to make sure he had a lift back home. Blackpool was a regular holiday destination for many of the families on the estate, though perhaps a less popular choice just for a night out, but Ted had no qualms about going further from home for more singing experience, sometimes even entering talent shows, winning and then bringing back whatever he earned. 'Ee ar our muv, I won this,' he'd say and hand over a small envelope. Hilda never knew if he was coming home or not, but she learned not to worry if his bed was empty in the morning.

'He never looked on the bad side of life,' says Ted's brother-in-law, Tony. 'No matter what you talked about, he'd always make it cheerful. It was as if all the troubles of the world could be on his shoulders but he was always out smiling. He never worried about a thing.'

One thing that Ted did learn early on was that even though sing-ing wasn't ever going to be his main job, it could still bring in some extra cash. He would often tell his dad: 'If you can get up and play an instrument or sing, you don't need any money when you go out 'cos they'll have a collection for you afterwards.' This was always the case in The Cora, where the crowd weren't shy about showing appreciation for great singers: it spoke volumes that there was always a collection for Ted whenever he got up to sing.

Mack the Knife

Ted remained close to all of his brothers – even as time marched on and they married, inevitably making their own lives outside the family home. He and Ernie were particularly tight, but so many of their scrapes and stories will remain untold – swallowed by the ravages of Alzheimer's in Ted's case and Ernie's early death from cancer in 2012.

Ernie probably knew more about the inner workings of Ted's mind than anyone else and their bond meant that he could see beyond his brother's cheery persona and ability to always see the good in any situation. Ernie's friends used to describe Ted as someone who could pick up any conversation and make it upbeat, but there was far more to him than that and his brother knew it. The frustration of not being able to make his passion a full-time job disheartened Ted as he got older and the opportunities slipped further away. He was most definitely ahead of his time and there was an honour in wanting to pursue it, but there was also the reality of responsibility and Ted knew he couldn't escape that; no one could.

But no matter how much real life kept elbowing its way in, Ted remained committed to music. Whenever a new record came out, he would go straight up to Paradise Street in West Bromwich and he'd return home with both the record and the sheet music, so that he could take it to the pub and ask the pianist to play it while he sang. One of his favourite record shops was Al Cooper's – he knew the owner and was always popping in whenever he could. In the cellars Al had all the old records from years back that he hadn't managed to sell; all the real classics had a little stamp on them – 2d – which was about the price of a pint of beer. So Ted would be down there for hours listening to Al's record stash, drinking tea and singing along – it was his ideal way to spend the day.

Playing music at Al's and at home took the edge off everything, even the fact he had very little money.

Every Saturday teatime, Ted would check the football pools, hoping to win, but never did, then go upstairs and get his record player out. Then it would start. He'd play the whole song through once, and then begin it again, but this time stopping after every line.

'Peg o' my heart, I'm calling...'

STOP

Then there would be a pause.

'Peg o' my heart, I'm calling, Peg o' my heart, I need you...'

STOP

And another pause.

He'd drive the household – especially Maurice – mad as he repeatedly stopped and started tracks, writing down the lyrics line by line so that he could learn them off by heart and sing the song all the way through over and over again. 'Christ's sakes, Big 'Un! If yam gunna play it, play it!' Maurice would shout. A new track would be learned every Saturday without fail, then Ted would get dressed up and go down to The Cora to showcase it. He had his finger on the pulse sending off for sheet music from America if he really liked something and never performed the same track twice. He'd always make sure he was the first to have all the latest songs, often sending his younger sister, Joyce, down to Woolworths with enough cash to buy a new record and a bag of broken biscuits as a reward for helping him out. In truth, the record player could have blown up the house, as at the time there were no plug sockets upstairs. That meant Ted running the cable to the record player through a light – essentially running a naked wire straight from the light fitting in the ceiling. It definitely took the idea of dying for his music to a whole new level. In fact, although Ted was known for helping out in any way he could, the one area that he was encouraged to keep away from was anything electrical. Maurice lived in fear of him trying to fix anything. If Ted became aware there was a problem, he would drop everything, roll up his sleeves and say to Hilda: 'Right, what do you need me to do?' But the whole house knew what a disaster he was and Malcolm, Gerry and Karen would hide behind the kitchen door, laughing as Ted got to grips with the job in hand. Often, if he didn't have a plug, he would just feed wires straight into the socket with a couple of matchsticks wedged in to stop them falling out. 'He's going to blow the bloody house up!' Maurice would shout, but Hilda thought he was a godsend.

It was around this time, in 1964, that Ted started hanging around the Pebble Mill studios in Birmingham, where the BBC was based. He met a lot of great people, all music lovers like him, all trying to turn their passion into something more. But there were three guys who Ted, now aged 28, met at this time and who would go on to transform his life: Ben Beards, Geoff Thompson and Fred Timmins. They were in similar situations to Ted – particularly Ben, who had a day job as a machinist at Wilkins and Mitchell in Darlaston, near Wednesbury, to provide for his wife and three young children. As well as working hard to bring home a decent wage, he also played the piano accordion and used his skill to earn extra cash and help pay his mortgage. Geoff, a 30-year-old drummer, joined him, and the two of them got a regular gig at a pub over in Bilston, where they were joined by Fred, a 22-year-old guitarist: they billed themselves as 'The Starliners'. Ben cleverly fitted his accordion with a microphone, allowing him to play the bass line and giving them a unique sound. Now and again he would get Fred to do a bit of singing, alongside playing his guitar, and this eventually led to a regular Thursday-night gig at the Friar Park Labour Club. The performances went down well but they didn't have the audience on their feet shouting for more. Fred's vocals were OK, but not standout, and they knew deep down that was holding them back – what they needed was a real star to belt out the lyrics. They were in luck one night when, during a break in their set, a handsome, well-dressed bloke with perfect hair walked up to the stage and asked: 'Can I sing wi ya, mate?'

It was Ted.

The band often had people coming up and wanting to sing, and it mostly didn't work as it was impossible to get a stranger to hit the right notes or sing in time. But there was something about Ted they thought was worth a go as he seemed to know his stuff.

'Do you know "Mack the Knife" in C?' he asked.

The band played the intro and Ted started the song flawlessly. The guys were stunned by the quality of his voice and his phrasing. By the time he had finished the whole audience was standing up and applauding – something that hadn't ever happened to them before.

Ben turned to Ted: 'You wanna job, mate?'

'Ar, go on. I'll 'av a go,' Ted replied.

'That was the night our lives changed for ever,' says Ben.

The following week or so, Ben booked a room in a pub to go through some songs with Ted, as well as buying a new portable organ to complete the band's sound. 'We only needed one crack at any song. He just got them – he always knew the words straight away, so things didn't take much practising, it was unreal,' says Ben.

After a couple of weeks of polishing their act, the band applied for a spot at the local Entertainers Club. It went down a storm. But there was one drawback – Ben felt Geoff the drummer was letting the band down, so he rang up Ronnie Cox, another drummer he knew, and he joined the band right away. It turned out that Ted and Ronnie knew each other – they'd grown up living a few streets apart, were the same age and had spent some of their earlier years getting into various scrapes and scuffles – and they got on like a house on fire. Ronnie was a real comic and Ted was constantly in hysterics at some of his jokes. The chemistry worked perfectly and no one doubted that Ted was having fun. Ronnie would just have to make a passing comment to Ted onstage and then the next thing he'd be falling about laughing hysterically.

For the next few months, the band kept the regular gig at the Friar Park Labour Club to polish their performances and to try out new songs. But they wanted bigger crowds, a higher bar, to challenge themselves with an audience that wasn't made up of locals who already knew and loved them. Finally, after perfecting their act, they were ready to up their game. Everything was now in sync for The Starliners to move on to bigger things. So they began to spread the net wider, and auditioned at different clubs around Wednesbury.

In the mid-1960s all the other bands were trying to copy The Beatles or The Shadows and were made up of kids ten years younger than Ted and the rest of the guys, who were all in their late twenties or early thirties. Sometimes the crowd didn't always appreciate the different style of music that The Starliners, with their broader musical influences, brought to the stage. But the rest of the time, their refusal to conform was their best asset, something that became obvious during one open audition night at Rugeley Miners Club. This night was the one time every month that the Midland's Entertainment Association – a group of social secretaries from pubs and clubs who were responsible for booking acts – were all in the same room. Once business had been taken care of, the night became the perfect shop window for them to witness potential talent first-hand. Bands would be queuing up to perform in front of the decision-makers in the hope of leaving an impression.

The Starliners were waiting by the side of the stage to go on. They were third in the line-up that night and the band on before them was a young group who had the audience on their feet. They also looked the part, with all the top gear – the best guitars, best drums, best speakers – and The Starliners stood watching them a bit lost for words as they belted out all The Beatles' and Shadows' numbers.

Despite feeling knocked by the huge reaction the youngsters received, Ted and the guys were ready as ever for their slot and, as soon as the stage was free, they set about getting everything in place. The previous band decided to wait in the wings and return the favour of watching their show. The only difference was that, as soon as Fred struck a chord, the other band started laughing and tried their best to distract Ted and the boys by shouting: 'What the hell is this, mate?' as they played 'Mack the Knife'. Ted kept time and they made it through to the end of the track without any slip-ups. However, despite the jeers from the other band, The Starliners had the last laugh.

The audience were on their feet dancing and after they'd finished, the applause for their set was the loudest of the day. 'We'll get a few bookings off this,' thought Ben. He was right. As the band walked offstage and made their way to the bar, they were stopped in their tracks by a host of agents, who surrounded them, desperate to book the boys for a whole number of gigs. Within an hour, they had taken sixty-four bookings, covering most of the clubs around Wednesbury and the Black Country. The other band left, expensive equipment in hand, without a single booking to their name.

For Ted this felt like a big step in the right direction. There was a real possibility of making this work in a more permanent way. Every single club they played at, without exception, booked them again; they had 100 per cent success rate. The Starliners were a tight unit and had developed their look as well as their sound. The band would wear scarlet jackets with black piping down the sleeves and collars, black trousers and a white shirt, apart from Ted who would go for a slightly different twist and sport a black jacket, a white shirt and bow tie. They were determined not to be one of those bands that just plugged in their guitars and wandered onto the stage. It wasn't just about the sound, it was about putting on a performance. They wanted to make a splash – if you could hook the audience within the first few seconds, you would have them for the rest of the night. If there was a curtain, it would be opened slowly and the band would strike up. Ted would then stride on to the stage, grab the mic and launch straight into the song. You could often hear the audience exclaim 'wow' as they got their first sighting of the slick outfits. The band could play everything for any generation: strict tempo, old-time dancing, Latin American, rock and roll – they covered it all.

The very thing they had been mocked for became their calling card, also helped by the fact that the 1960s craze for ballroom dancing had hit fever pitch and there were very few bands who could cater to that as most were beginning a love affair with rock. The brilliance of the music favoured by Ted and the boys was that it lent itself beautifully to quicksteps, foxtrots or waltzes. The Starliners would simply adjust the tempo and it became great music for all occasions – the dance floor was full to capacity at every gig and the audience, whatever the age, couldn't get enough. Word soon spread around the Midlands about Teddy Mac and The Starliners – they never had to audition again.

The group was ambitious and being creative was something Ted excelled at. He thought about every note, every movement, what they would all wear and even how they would stand on the stage in front of the audience – all for maximum impact and designed to put on the best show possible. Sometimes the band would tinker with a song so that they could put their own spin on a classic and really bring the house down. All of this came as second nature to Ted, but he had to admit he didn't really have a head for business. That fell to Ben, who took over the day-to-day running of things and dealt with the bookings and the fair splitting of the profits. The booking requests started coming from further afield and they had clubs in Manchester, Leeds and Liverpool asking them to do gigs. They all agreed to put a limit on how far they were prepared to travel as they had day jobs, so they settled on a 40-mile radius as the maximum distance.

By this time the band began to rehearse regularly in a room in St Giles Church Hall in Willenhall. A group called The 'N Betweens used to rehearse in the room before them and as the two groups were swapping over they'd usually have a chat about which gigs they were doing and what was coming up. 'In later years that band went massive,' says Ben. 'It was Noddy Holder and they became the Seventies glam-rock superstars Slade.'

Christmas was a bumper time for The Starliners – they were booked practically every night throughout December. 'I don't know how we did it,' says Ben. 'We used to do about twenty-six or twenty-seven nights that month. We'd get home around two o'clock in the morning, go to bed, and be up for work at seven, then get home around 5 p.m., have a quick nap for an hour, pack up and then be at another club for seven the next night. But the money we made was unbelievable. I reckon in today's money we'd be getting around £1,500 for each of those nights.

'We were beginning to get really well known by this time. Whenever we did a gig, we'd turn up and often find "House Full" notices on the outside of venues,' he adds.

The Starliners were beginning to acquire a huge following and Ted was always popular with the ladies. 'We used to have to sneak him out by the back door to the car park sometimes because of all the women who were after him at the end of the night,' says Ben. 'You'd be onstage and you'd see all these women throwing their telephone numbers on the stage. But he hardly went with any of them. I think he was seeing someone at the time. But the groupies could be too much sometimes – they'd be literally throwing themselves at you. It wasn't pretty.'

As with everything to do with his romantic life, Ted kept his cards close to his chest. The band suspected he was seeing someone, but his friends and family had no idea that he was also still in touch with Iris.

'Well, after we split up, we still kept in touch,' she says. 'It wasn't an affair as such. We'd meet for a coffee and a cake up West Bromwich or wherever and he'd tell me what he was up to – where he was singing, what songs he was doing and all that, the band and everything. He wouldn't stop talking. You know, after we split up he said to me, "If yow ever need to talk, I'll meet you at one o'clock on Saturday by the clock in West Bromwich." We could go twelve months without seeing each other and have no contact and then I'd pop up to West Brom on a Saturday and he'd be there waiting by the clock. We did that for years and years – that was before phones. I would just turn up at one o'clock to see if he was around and he'd usually be stood there waiting. At one o'clock. It went on for years.'

Says Ben: 'I remember another night at the Bloxwich Memorial club. This club was one of the biggest clubs in the area and all the top-name national acts used to play there. Mac [Ted] had them eating out of his hand. Not only was he a great singer, but by now he had become a brilliant frontman too, with a great line of patter with the audience. We'd overrun a bit that night and towards the end of the show the audience were getting up to catch their last buses home. That's when Mac began to sing the classic "Look Down That Lonesome Road". Everyone stopped dead in their tracks. There was thunderous applause. I'll never forget that. One of the most memorable nights in the band I had.'

He continues: 'A few weeks after that we had a call from the owner of Walsall Football Club asking if we could do the opening of their new social club. We were well known with the football club and had already done gigs there. Ken Dodd [great music-hall entertainer and stand-up comic famous for his buck teeth and 'tickling sticks', i.e. feather dusters] was top of the bill and The Starliners were booked to support him.' Ben remembers it as the greatest night of his musical career: 'We went on first for an hour or so, and there were a couple of local acts after us. At around 10 p.m. Ken Dodd came on and did about two hours non-stop. He had the place in stitches and tore it apart. We backed him for his songs "Happiness" and "Tears for Souvenirs".' All the money that was raised that night went to a local charity – even Ken Dodd waived his fee. 'He was a lovely bloke, Doddy was,' says Ben. 'There's some people that look down on the public, but everyone was the same to Ken – he was great.' The following morning back at Kent Road, when all the kids woke up, they were excited to find the lounge full of tickling sticks that Ted had brought home from the show; proudly taking them to school to show their friends.

After the Ken Dodd gig, The Starliners were inundated with bookings, there was a real momentum to the group and, for the first time since that very early outing onstage at the Friar Park Labour Club, it seemed that Ted's lifelong dream of making it big was finally coming true. That's when the band received a call from an agent saying he wanted them to do a tour of the US Army bases in Germany. It was a massive gig and they would be on tour for weeks. Ted couldn't believe they would be going abroad – the furthest he'd travelled was to Blackpool. This was life-changing and he told the family as soon as he had the news. No one could believe that 'our Ted' was going so far away. For Hilda, who had been so delighted that all her children had chosen to stay near home, this was exciting and devastating in equal measure.

But Ted's hopes were dashed before they could even make plans. Ben called a meeting to discuss the opportunity and Ted could tell immediately there was something wrong by everyone's long faces. They definitely weren't the expressions of men who had just been told they were going to Germany to do the thing they loved most.

It was Ben who was given the job of delivering the crushing blow – they couldn't go. The rest of them had day jobs, mortgages to pay and families to look after – they weren't footloose like Ted and their responsibilities kept them tied down at home. It was a crushing blow for Ted and a sobering moment for the band – they knew they were holding him back. The good times stopped rolling and it didn't take long for the rot to set in, especially when the tight-knit group made the mistake of letting others in.

By 1968, Ronnie's dad, Jack, had begun to help out with setting up the occasional gig, as well as driving them to and from venues. It helped relieve some of the pressure on Ben, who had a wife and kids to get back for. The problem was that once Jack had a formal role with the band, the power slowly went to his head. He started acting as if he ran the show – and that included telling Ted what to do. It was clear that Ted wasn't too happy with the new order but Ben didn't want to rock the boat; after all, Jack was giving them a hand lugging all the equipment around and driving them about. 'He was a great guy but he could sometimes be too outspoken,' says Ben.

It all came to a head one Wednesday night at Woods Social Club in Wednesbury. It had been a typical knockout gig for The Starliners and the crowd had gone wild. After a couple of drinks at the end of the night, they were all packing up the equipment. Ted was joking around with the rest of the lads when, by accident as he was unplugging the microphone from the stand, he dropped it. 'That's when it happened,' says Ben. 'Jack went ballistic at Ted. The microphone belonged to the band and Jack just laid into him – telling him he needed to be more careful. But he went completely over the top towards Ted.' This pushed Ted over the edge. He wasn't being spoken to like that, no matter who Jack was, and he told him in no uncertain terms where he could stick his mic.

Then he picked up his coat.

'Bugger this. I'm off,' he said and walked out.

Jack was immediately fired and Ben tried to persuade their frontman to come back. But it was too late – as far as Ted was concerned, the damage had been done, and the band never heard from him again. He might have wanted fame and fortune and the chance to sing onstage every night, but he wasn't being spoken to like that. Some called it principled, Hilda saw it as Ted being his usual stubborn self; Iris saw it as him sabotaging something he felt deep down would implode anyway. Either way, although Ben was devastated and hoped Ted would cool down after a few weeks, he also wasn't about to beg him to stay. Eventually, another singer got in touch about joining them, Ted was replaced and the band went on to perform for another twenty years.

Ben admits it was never quite the same again:

'I just wish I'd asked him to come back. Looking back, that's the one thing I regret. He was great. I can honestly say – and I'm not just saying this – that there's no one else I'd rather be in a band with. He was a great bloke – with everybody. Everybody loved him. He was never a big head – to be honest, I don't think he realized just how good he was. He never planned for anything – whatever he had that day was what he was happy with. He really loved his life, you know.'

After a few months, Ben heard that Ted was doing Saturday nights at The Cora, so he went down to see him. Ted was doing what he loved best – running the show, getting people on the stage to sing, as well as doing the occasional spot himself. The place was packed out and as soon as Ben walked in, Ted flashed him his biggest smile. Never one to hold grudges he was glad to see his old mate. Ben had actually planned to ask Ted to come back that night, but he could see he was in his element and so he left it – between the two of them there was a lot of male pride at stake. Ben readily acknowledged that the band was nothing before Ted joined, that he was one of a kind and just had that 'something'. The band made a lot of money; Ben certainly found that his wife's reservations fell by the wayside once she realized it had paid for their house. But Ted didn't have that kind of responsibility outside the band – he very much lived each day as it came and didn't expect anything to last.

'For years I always wondered what happened to him,' says Ben. 'It was just when I was watching the TV last September when that video came on of him singing in the car. I nearly fell off my chair. I shouted to my wife, "Bloody hell! That's Ted McDermott! That's Teddy Mac!"

'Honestly, I always thought he would go on to bigger and better things. He was world class – there was just something about him. You know, I really hoped he would make it someday. Well, he has really – it's just that he's 80, though…'

Tap Your Troubles Away

It was 1968, Ted had left The Starliners and was back to doing his Saturday-night gig at The Cora and the occasional night at different clubs, but it wasn't regular work and he wasn't making as much money as when he'd been in the band, plus he didn't have his own transport, meaning he was limited to where he could travel. He had lots of odd jobs during the day to ensure he could pay Hilda his board, and there was no doubt that Maurice and Hilda loved still having him at home, but they would also pass many a night sitting in the front room, each in their respective armchairs, wondering when he would settle down.

Of course, the younger siblings still lived at home too, but some of them were still at school, unlike Ted, who was in his thirties and seemingly lost. He'd gone from being at the top of his game, singing in one of the most popular bands in the Midlands, to making ends meet with irregular jobs and irregular hours. Maurice would be reading the paper and Hilda would be sewing something for one of the many grandchildren they were welcoming into the family and she couldn't help but wonder when, or even if, she would be doing the same thing for Ted. He might have been following his passion, but as far as they were concerned, he was also their firstborn, 32 years old and living at home with no car, no girlfriend and no regular job. His brothers and sisters were all settling down around him and he seemed to be, at best, stuck, at worst, going backwards. On top of this, Ted began to smoke like a chimney, which drove his dad mad, as he thought it was a total waste of money.

Ted's younger brother Fred (now married with a good job as a builder and his own car) came up with a brilliant solution to the transport problem and decided he would drive him to the open-mic nights. It meant Ted could not only save money on getting there (because Fred refused payment), but also earn the maximum possible. Despite leaving The Starliners, Ted was still in high demand and knew he had to capitalize on that. But what soon became apparent to Fred was that Ted wasn't charging nearly enough for a gig. He set the price as low as six or seven pounds for his booking, when he was worth double that – both in terms of talent *and* compared to the competition.

Ted was never pushy when it came to getting onstage – more often than not he'd let other singers go on before him, which often meant he'd be last on the list. But if the compère was taking too much time warming up the crowd, Ted would sometimes end up not singing at all. In reality, he needed a manager to deal with the business side so that he could just get on with the singing, but Ted also wanted to be his own man. The family were all still proud of Ted's ability to wow an audience. Fred could see it everywhere he went, especially when he drove him around to any auditions and gigs and there would often be a queue around the block when Ted was booked to sing.

So Fred appointed himself as Ted's new manager and was in charge of the bookings, driving him around to the many 'shop windows' where entertainers would perform for the club secretaries. He initially started charging the clubs six or seven pounds for Ted to do a spot, but then when he saw the number of secretaries queuing up to book him, he decided to up it. 'How much yam charging for the Mill Lane Club?' said one.

'Ten quid, mate,' said Fred.

'Ten quid – that's a bloody lot, ay it?' the guy replied.

'Ah, well. He's worth it, ay he? Why yam standing in the queue for if you don't wanna pay it?' said Fred.

'We'll pay it. Will he do two twenty-minute spots?' said the guy.

Fred became a shrewd negotiator and decided that planning was everything. He made friends with all the entertainment secretaries at every venue, bought them a pint as Ted performed and wowed the crowd, and then, once they were bowled over, he would land the killer punch and tell them Ted's fee had doubled and he wouldn't be going anywhere for under £20 if they wanted him to come back. He would have it all lined up perfectly for when Ted finished his set, handing him a drink and filling him in on what to say when they approached him for another booking. They both agreed that Ted had to ask for £22 and accept £18 when he would get bartered down, which was much better than the measly £9 he was charging.

Fred felt happy with the fact that his big brother would finally get paid what he deserved. It was about damn time as far as he was concerned.

But things didn't go to plan. It was after one of Ted's legendary performances, with everything nicely lined up for him to request the new higher fee, that the entertainment secretary Jimmy came straight over to congratulate Ted and ask if they could book him again for six months' time.

'What sort of money are you looking at, mate?' said Jimmy.

'Nine quid,' said Ted without even blinking.

Fred put down his pint, walked straight out of the club and went back to his car. Despite feeling grateful for all Fred's hard work in raising the price and being bowled over by how much the queuing crowd was prepared to pay to hear him sing, Ted felt he just couldn't ask people to pay double the price they'd paid before. He knew it made perfect business sense and that, in order to sing for a living, this was what he had to do, but he just couldn't. 'Our Ted would pour his heart and soul out on that stage,' says Fred. 'But he was so daft when it came down to the hard cash. He just wanted to sing for free!'

Fred was livid. His brother was a law unto himself and he was sick of seeing Ted sell himself short. Ted came strolling out of the club, looking for Fred.

'Get in the car, our Big. I'm gunna drop you off now and I'm never tekin' you anywhere else again. You gotta paddle your own boat.'

'What's up, our Fred?'

'What's bloody up? What's bloody up? You working your bloody guts out and me driving all this way to get you some bloody money and you won't bloody ask for what you're worth. That's what's up. How much do you think yam gunna make in the world if yow don't start bloody asking for it?'

He wasted no time in reminding him that he needed cash to look the part and also take some of the strain away from Hilda – who still washed and ironed his shirts when he could pay for them to be laundered if he had money. 'That's where the bloody money is!' shouted Fred, pointing back to the club. 'Yow singing! And yow won't bloody ask for it!'

He dropped him off and never took him again.

After this Ted made his own way around doing gigs, but although he was still a popular choice for many of the clubs, the fact that he didn't have a car meant he was limited to how far he could travel. The brothers made up but Fred despaired and, privately, so did the rest of the family. The singing was all he had, so why couldn't he really make the most of it? Hilda was also preoccupied by the fact that, since Iris, there really hadn't been anyone special in Ted's life.

One weekend, a few friends from The Cora came to the house to try and persuade Ted to come out with them to a house party hosted by a well-known local musician in Dudley. Eventually, they sweet-talked him into tagging along. He was glad he did. It was there he met

Janet Cann. Janet had been involved in showbiz since she was a child. Her dad played the accordion and encouraged both Janet, who sang, and her sister, who played the vibraphone, to go onstage. But all that Janet wanted to do was sing in a band. She was ten years younger than Ted, but the fact she was a performer instantly made her intriguing and they talked for most of the night. They agreed to meet up later that week when Ted had a gig on. It was on this first date, as the band struck up and Ted opened his mouth to sing, that Janet instantly fell in love with his voice.

Janet had a day job working as a secretary at the then ATV in Birmingham, but, like Ted, she performed at dancehalls around the Midlands, singing with the Don Trent Dance Band. They loved the same music and eventually decided to bring their shared sound together by setting up a vocal duo – 'Mac and Jan' – doing gigs around the Midlands, with Janet's dad taking over Fred's role and driving them back and forth. Things quickly became serious and Ted took her home to meet the family almost immediately. Like Iris, Janet came from a small family and marvelled at the closeness of Ted's as they bantered in the kitchen and finished each other's sentences. But, despite all Ted's affection and his love of romantic gestures, she would complain to friends that they didn't actually ever go on a date – they either sat in watching TV with his family or went down to the club and spent the evening with a big crowd. Romance seemed in short supply as far as Janet was concerned, especially as Ted would often talk of 'beautiful' Iris and how she'd got married – perhaps not ideal courting behaviour when you're out to impress someone new! 'Looking back on it now, we were both nursing broken hearts. I'd just came out of a relationship and it was obvious he was still in love with Iris,' says Janet.

Janet also noticed that Ted seemed to have an agitated energy he couldn't control that manifested as mood swings. They dated for two years until she felt forced to end things. In her mind there was no plan, no romance – only singing. Ted didn't seem interested in their future together and she wanted some stability. In that whole two years she didn't even know what he did for a job during the day or whether she was coming or going. She just wanted a normal relationship and felt there was only room for one love in his life – and it was singing. 'We'd walk around the park singing together, then sit on a bench planning what we'd sing at the next do we'd go to,' says Janet. 'But then he'd just come round unexpectedly some nights saying we had a gig and we had to leave right there and then. I just got fed up with it.'

Yet again, Hilda and Maurice found themselves quietly discussing Ted's inability to settle down. It was as if he was holding himself back, and the sad thing was that, deep down, Ted knew it, too. He was melancholic and it was difficult for him to find the joy he so desperately wanted. His relationship with Janet became a casualty of that – on the surface she was perfect and she even shared his musical passion – but he just couldn't get it together.

The next few years were dark times for Ted, and the family worried about him. He still did the occasional gig at The Cora, but other than that, Hilda had no idea where he worked or what he did half the time. He started wasting his money on soft bets and endless games of pinball that paid out £10 or £15 a time, and he was losing himself day by day. He would spend whole afternoons sitting in front of the TV, puffing on a cigarette. Hilda and Maurice retreated to traditional roles – she fussed and tried to make everything OK and Maurice became irritated and unsympathetic with his son's fall from grace. As far as he was concerned, he'd had a damn good life and had let it slip through his fingers. Ted's brothers and sisters varied in their sympathy – unimpressed by his gambling and the fact he spent the mornings in bed while they all grafted. Hilda was ever-protective: 'Yam remember! You wanna stop and think.

He used to turn all of his wages over when he first started work so most of you lot could eat!' She was still proud of him and wouldn't put up with any criticism.

In typical Ted fashion he always stepped up in a crisis and there was no bigger test than the death of his beloved father. In many ways Maurice led a textbook life for the times – he had worked hard all his adult years in a steady job, married the love of his life and given his children every opportunity he could. He had lived in the same house for nearly thirty years, brought home a regular wage and enjoyed putting the world to rights down at the local club over a pint with the friends he'd known since he was young. He needed very little in order to enjoy life, except to have Hilda by his side, which is exactly what he had until the end. Mercifully for Maurice (but heartbreakingly for Hilda), when the end came, it was quick.

Maurice hadn't been feeling himself for a few months – he was exhausted with grumbling stomach pains that wouldn't go away. He went back and forth to the doctor and was given various types of medicine for the cramps but nothing seemed to work. He was coming in from work, collapsing in his chair, and going straight to sleep without much appetite or enthusiasm for anything. He began to lose weight and look drawn, and Hilda was beside herself – no matter what she cooked he wouldn't eat and that wasn't like Maurice at all. Eventually, Hilda took him back to the doctor's and they referred him to the hospital for an exploratory operation the following month. The day arrived and she got up early to pack his overnight bag and lay out fresh clothes, just as she had done every day of their married life. They said their goodbyes and she waved him off from the front-room window. Maurice told her to stay at home while one of the boys drove him to the hospital. He reasoned there was no point in her pacing about there when she could be in the comfort of her own home. Hilda knew that one of the kids would come by as soon as there was any news and she wasn't that worried. It was only a routine operation to see what was causing the pain, after all.

She took her mind off things by cleaning and cooking, while Maurice was taken into theatre by their daughter Jane, who decided to stay and wait for news. After what seemed like no time at all a nurse ushered her and the rest of the siblings into a side room to tell them how things had gone. It wasn't good news – they had opened Maurice up to find the cause and seen that he was riddled with stomach cancer. There was nothing to be done apart from closing him back up and letting the family say their goodbyes.

It all happened so fast and someone had to go and break the news to Hilda, who was in so much shock that she couldn't get to the hospital in time to see her beloved husband. In the end Maurice never did come round from the operation and everyone knew the end was near. As Jane says: 'You just know when it's the last moments.'

They all knew it was bleak, but believing strongly that while there's life, there's hope, they all rallied round. Ted decided the best thing he could do was put on his usual cheery front; he came breezing into the ward and went straight to the top of the bed. He stroked the hair back from Maurice's face and kissed him on the forehead whispering: 'Yam alright, Mac.' And just like that, Maurice died. All the children were sure that he let go at that moment because he mistook Ted's hand for Hilda's and thought she was there, saying a final goodbye. He was 63.

Everyone was shattered; it was like the heart had been ripped out of the family. Hilda was inconsolable. She had no idea what to do without Maurice – they had spent thirty-eight years as a couple, seeing through the good and the bad times. Knowing that his body was at the hospital was heartbreaking as they had barely spent a night apart, but the children all stayed with her. They couldn't help but be terrified by how diminished she already seemed, averting her gaze from Maurice's empty chair in the front room.

Ted was determined not to show his upset and didn't shed a tear, not in front of the others anyway. His motto was: 'It dow matter if you're going to a wedding or a funeral – hold yer head up! Dow let 'em see! Dow let 'em see!' Ernie and Colin on the other hand cried non-stop in those early days. Maurice was buried in Heath Lane Cemetery in a plot big enough for two and the house was heavy with grief, long after the funeral and wake, which was attended by people far and wide. He was loved – whether you'd met him down the pub, watched him sing or worked alongside him, he was known as a true gent. People said they didn't make them like him any more and that is most definitely how Hilda wanted him to be remembered.

Ted found living with the sadness hard but when an advertisement for a job as an entertainer at Butlin's came up, he was completely torn. On the one hand, he felt sad at the thought of leaving Hilda, on the other he knew that Maurice wouldn't have wanted him to wallow for ever, and it was time to move on. Hilda didn't really leave the house as much as she used to. She was seeing less of her friends, and had recently been diagnosed with diabetes, which began to take its toll on her. Ted knew that seeing her fade away bit by bit every day would kill him, so being away was a way of pretending things hadn't changed.

It made financial sense too, as there would be free food and board, which meant he would save money on living and travel expenses. He wrestled with the dilemma for days and, in the end, after talking to Hilda, he decided to apply. Once he'd posted the application, Ted tried to put it out of his mind, because he knew that if he got the job then his life would change for ever. There'd be no more travelling for miles to small gigs by night and doing odd jobs he hated by day. Instead, he would perform in front of a huge audience every single night and he would live alongside other performers who were learning their craft. But he'd also be miles away from home, living alone for the first time. Although he'd spent time in the Army, it wasn't far away and

Ted had popped back to see his family every weekend. Working at Butlin's would be completely different: he would be miles and miles away from home – plus, whenever he came home, he'd be confronted with the fact that Maurice was no longer there.

Ted kept his application to himself as he didn't want to tempt fate and he had no idea how long the process would take. Butlin's was *the* place to go on holiday with your family and prided itself on having 'something for everyone'. Ted knew getting the job was a long shot, but, somehow, just applying made him realize how desperate he was for a change. A few weeks later, he got the letter telling him that he had succeeded and would be posted to Barry Island, in Wales. This was the start of a brand-new chapter and, after years of doing the same thing, suddenly he had no idea what was in store for him.

Ted and Hilda didn't really discuss the job in the run-up to him leaving, as she couldn't stand the thought of seeing him go so soon after Maurice's death. However, she also remembered all those late-night conversations about Ted and how worried they'd been, and she knew Maurice would be urging him to grab the chance of change with both hands. There were lots of goodbyes and everyone was sad to see Ted leave; it was difficult, but it was also exciting.

The Butlin's holiday camp stood on a headland overlooking the beach and the small town and featured all the usual Butlin's sights – the Pig & Whistle Pub, the Gaiety Theatre, ballroom, tennis courts, snooker tables, shops and dining room. There was plenty to see. The camp itself was a picturesque seaside resort, with uninterrupted views of the beautiful Welsh coast. Ted couldn't believe it when he arrived – everywhere smelled of the sea and there wasn't a factory in sight.

Once he had settled in he realized that living away from home meant he had to make friends, and quickly, so he set about getting to know as many people as possible. One of the first people he met on the camp was Brian Ward – a.k.a. Wardie. He was a comedian and compère for many of the shows at the Gaiety Theatre, and a big friendly northerner who wouldn't be seen without his tie.

Wardie's route into showbiz began when he was working, like Ted, in the Army. He was posted in Oman at the same time as comedian Bob Monkhouse was sent there to entertain the troops. His job was to accompany Monkhouse to and from the show and it was on one of these nights that Wardie got talking to him about how he too could get onstage. He boldly took Bob to one side and asked him: 'So, Bob, if I wanted to do what you do, what's the best way I could do it?'

'Butlin's,' said Monkhouse.

A few years later Monkhouse was doing a show at Butlin's when he spotted Wardie in the audience. In the middle of his patter, he stopped.

'Wardie?! What are you doing here?'

'I'm a Red now,' Wardie said.

They became great friends and would always have a drink together whenever Monkhouse did a gig at any Butlin's where Wardie happened to be working.

Meanwhile, in Barry Island, as part of the on-site entertainment, the Redcoats would put on a weekly panto for the kids and Ted was in his element. Wardie would always play the baddie, scaring all the kids and screaming: 'I'm gonna kill you!' as he crept around the stage. Ted's role was to come out of the woods dressed as Robin Hood in green tights, shouting in his broad Black Country accent: 'Yam kids come with me. Yam safe now.' He loved being the one to rescue them and threw himself into the role with great passion.

The routine that Ted so badly craved was there right from the first day and the job as a Redcoat began from the moment he got up at 7 a.m. and went to breakfast. In a way it was the perfect job for a grieving son who didn't want to deal with his feelings, because he had to be in character at all times. His role was to make people laugh and to make them happy – two things Ted had always been good at.

After breakfast there would be time to chat to the guests and get to know them, competitions to organize, bingo, the donkey derby, *It's a Knockout* style games, sports days, as well as performing daytime and evening shows. Everyone loved Ted, guests and workers alike, and he quickly gained a reputation as a hard worker.

As ever, Ted managed to perform whenever he could and was often found singing in the Pig & Whistle as well as doing shows in the Gaiety Theatre. Billy Butlin used to boast that the stage of the Gaiety was bigger than the London Palladium – by a mighty 6 inches! Each night it would be packed, with more than 2,000 people watching the show. It was a dream come true for Ted to be singing in a venue that size. The enormity of it got him every time and he would often imagine what his dad would have made of the whole thing.

Being that bit older than a lot of the Redcoats, Ted was quite the catch among the staff and holiday-goers alike. He discovered a new-found freedom and confidence there. Perhaps it was the liberation of being far away from home and knowing that trouble wouldn't follow him down to the local club, or maybe it was just the confidence of being a man in his mid-thirties. Either way, the stories of what went on are Ted's alone.

Whenever Ted had a day off, he would make his way back to the Midlands to see the family, no matter how brief it was. But every time he left he felt torn between looking after Hilda and the responsibility for the household and going out there and following his dream – which would in turn bring in much-needed cash and make Hilda proud.

At the end of the 1974 season at Barry Island, Ted and Wardie decided to go to London and look for jobs in showbiz. They found some digs in Leytonstone on the outskirts – Ted having no idea about the city that he had just found himself in – and set about trying to find work. The Big Smoke was *the* place to be to find fame and fortune. The problem was that they needed an Equity card (proof of membership of

Equity, the trade union for performing artists), which Ted didn't have, so the whole trip was a disaster and put him firmly back at square one in terms of his chances of West End fame. This meant it was back to the Midlands, still searching for work, and doing whatever factory job he could find at the time.

But his luck was about to change. Come October, Ted was invited to audition for the Butlin's Tour Show.

The tour show was a shop window to help promote the entertainment programme at Butlin's camps around the country. During intervals, the tour manager and his wife would walk around the audience handing out leaflets and chatting to people about Butlin's holidays, trying to persuade them to book up. It was a huge sales event. Well, that was the plan anyway. In reality, the lack of any decent budget meant that it was very much done on the cheap, with the acts doing their best to put on a knock-out two-and-half-hour show to various audiences around the country without much investment.

The audition for the Butlin's Tour Show took place at Butlin's Minehead – a resort in Somerset, south-west England. Entertainers from across the country auditioned and one of these was Barry Bennett – a comedian and impressionist in his mid-twenties who was already well known on the entertainment circuit in the Midlands.

A couple of days before he was due to drive down to Minehead from the Midlands, he received a call from his agent asking if he could pick up Ted McDermott, who was also auditioning for the show. Barry lived on the Hyde Road Estate in Wednesbury – about three miles from Kent Road, where Ted was again living. So, the day before the audition, Barry drove round to Kent Road in his Rover 2000, waited outside Ted's house in Friar Park and honked his horn. Ted came out of the house with a brown suitcase, wearing his smart blue suit, and with Hilda waving him off at the window. Despite both of them being in the business and living not far from each other, the two had never met before, but they soon got on, sharing stories about entertaining on the drive down to Minehead. When they arrived, they were both given chalets to stay in and told the auditions and rehearsals were the next day in the Gaiety Theatre on the camp.

But when they got to the theatre, everything was in complete disarray. The organist was late, there was no music and nobody had brought any of the uniforms they were meant to be performing in. Ted turned to Barry and, under his breath laughing, said: 'This is a shambles.' Barry agreed.

Like most people who had yet to see Ted come to life onstage, Barry had no idea how good he would be and just assumed he was another newcomer about to be thrown in at the deep end. Barry says: 'Offstage, he didn't seem like an entertainer and I remember thinking to myself, "This guy hasn't got a clue what he's doing."' As they watched all the other acts nervously go onstage, Ted was relaxed and chatting away with everyone. But as soon as he stepped onto that stage he left no doubt about how polished he was as a performer. Everyone else climbed onto the stage and gave a little talk about their act – but not Ted. He simply walked on when the music started and began singing. He didn't need to explain to anybody what his act was, *he* was his act. One of the things that stood out for those in the know was that Ted had the most tremendous phraseology and the ability to sing one sentence in one breath (something only the most accomplished singers like Jim Reeves and Frank Sinatra can do). There was no breathing between words as modern singers tend to do and it gave Ted's voice that unique sound that everyone loved. The other thing that made him stand out from the rest was his understated stage presence and the fact that he didn't move around – he could work on a three-foot square of carpet. It was all about his gestures and that was very, very Sinatra.

After the auditions, the final team was selected and it was no surprise that Ted had made the cut, along with Barry, Dave Thomas as another comedian, Glenn Martin on the drums, Steve, a keyboard player, and Emma, a female vocalist (who was also to be the girlfriend of Glenn Martin).

At the start of the tour, the Butlin's uniforms that had been provided for the group were all the wrong size and Dave Thomas refused to wear his, claiming it looked 'a bloody sack'. Instead, Ted, Dave and Barry wore the cabaret suits they'd brought from home, while the rest wore the uniform. Having spent a lifetime looking the part, Ted wasn't about to compromise his style for anyone, even if it meant going against the dress code. He had never really conformed and he wasn't about to start now.

There's No Business Like Show Business

The group were thrown together and were expected to put on a show that highlighted the ultimate Butlin's experience. But it was hit and miss at first – they were all very different and there was no one taking the reins. After a few rehearsals, they decided they'd test out the show at the Pig & Whistle – to their surprise, it was a great success. But the gang soon realized they really needed another act to fill the show. Glenn Martin – the drummer of the group – announced that he was quite good with a crossbow and suggested that they create a new circus-style act – Egor and Gallia, The Magic Duo – that would bring an element of peril and drama. Glenn would go backstage and turn into the wild Egor, while the female vocalist, Emma, would transform into the exotic Gallia – a Russian siren. The audience were none the wiser, as they were completely unrecognizable. Gallia would stand in front of a blackboard with Pepsi cans or apples balanced on her head and a blindfolded Egor (guided by the sound of Gallia's voice) would launch arrows at these items. Although the audience didn't know it, Egor had a monocle within the blindfold and a small hole so that he could see before he fired off his life-threatening arrows.

It was a dangerous act that always drew gasps from the audience. Ted refused to compère, as he didn't think it was safe, and spent the whole time feeling terrified that someone would end up with an arrow in their forehead. He left it to Dave or Barry to get the audience going and instead concentrated on his own act. It turned out he was right to be anxious as one night Glenn quietly whispered to Barry: 'I can't see anything.'

Barry stalled the show a bit, again asking for quiet from the audience. You could hear a pin drop in the theatre.

'Ten, nine, eight…'

Again Egor whispered: 'I can't see anything.'

It turned out that the room was so smoky, Egor's monocle had fogged up inside his blindfold – he was totally blind and had a room full of people believing that was the whole point.

'Ladies and gentleman, we do require complete silence for this act…' said Barry, stalling again.

'Hold on – I think I can see now,' whispered Egor.

Everyone on the stage was terrified. Gallia later said that her life flashed before her very eyes and Barry kept his tightly shut as Egor fired the arrow straight at her head. When they all managed to look up, the Pepsi can on top of Gallia's head had split in two – but so had the top of her actual head – and she had rivers of blood pouring down her face.

'Just a little scratch, ladies and gentlemen, just a little scratch…' announced Barry as Gallia was guided off the stage, cursing Egor as she went behind the curtain and nearly fainted. They were all professionals, however, and, after a quick clean-up backstage, the show went on, going down as one of the best nights of the tour.

The tour travelled around the country for a number of weeks – but it was so badly organized that it made no geographical sense. One day they would be down south and the next day they'd find themselves having to go back up north to another theatre, only to have to come all the way down again. Initially they all travelled around in a minibus together, staying at whatever digs they could find. But because of the poor planning, some of the group decided to bring their own cars and caravans as a way of guaranteeing themselves somewhere to stay.

Dave Thomas brought along his caravan, which Ted and Barry stayed in when they could. Ted and Dave had the beds, while Barry always slept on the floor. Glenn and his girlfriend Emma (Egor and Gallia) also had their own trailer and they would all drive in a convoy in order to make sure they arrived together as an act. Although he wasn't exactly used to living like a king on tour, even Ted was shocked the first time he saw the size of Dave's caravan parked outside one of the venues – it was so tiny that he had no idea how they would all fit inside. But any concerns soon disappeared when it became clear they were all determined to have as much fun as possible.

Glenn's trailer was literally that – a trailer attached to the back of the car. The rest of the group didn't believe that Glenn and his girlfriend would actually be able to sleep in it. But sure enough, when they dropped open the back of it there was indeed a mattress and some blankets. Then out popped a duck and a dog – two pets that Glenn and his girlfriend always brought along with them whenever they went touring. It was bizarre to say the least!

The tour was a steep learning curve and anything but glamorous – they certainly weren't living the high life and the money was poor – in fact, some weeks they wouldn't get paid at all. Often they didn't shower for days on end, and they had to dream up all kinds of tricks to make sure they were fed. Dave used to take Ted and Barry to the local Co-op and ask for as many food samples as they could, playing up to the fact that they were Butlin's Redcoats living on the breadline. They soon found themselves with handfuls of cheese, black pudding and whatever other bits they could get their hands on, which they would carefully smuggle back to the trailer, trying not to drop anything along the way. This would keep them going throughout the day and then in the evenings, the club would either feed them or they would have to grab a packet of crisps from behind the bar. In the mornings they would each take turns going to houses to beg for eggs or bacon so they could have something to eat.

The group would often park up and sleep in the car parks of the clubs or theatres in which they were playing. Because it was winter, they'd find themselves cracking open the ice on buckets of water so that they could shave. A hot bath and clean clothes felt like distant memories, but they didn't care – there would be plenty of time for showers later. For now, they were free and living their dreams: it didn't get any better than that.

The rest of the family didn't hear the end of it when Ted came home – if they hadn't all been so close then it might have caused trouble between them. After all, they were the ones looking after Hilda, doing her shopping and making sure she had her medication, when suddenly Ted would stroll in, make Hilda laugh and then disappear again for another few weeks, leaving the rest of them to cope with the daily grind.

The tour carried on relentlessly, taking them all over the country. Although they were always welcome, some crowds could be tricky to manage. One of the worst nights was a booking to play a theatre on the outskirts of London.

It was a huge club, with a massive audience; the place was packed full of people sitting at hard tables and chairs, shouting and jeering for the acts to come on to the stage and get going. Barry had just finished his act and Ted was about to walk on to start his when, all of a sudden, a heavily pregnant woman who was walking in front of the stage was kicked in the stomach by a man. All hell broke loose and it was the biggest fight either Ted or Barry had ever seen. Luckily for them the stage was five feet off the ground, meaning the audience, who were now in the midst of a full-blown riot, forgot that the acts were onstage.

Ted and the rest of the gang dragged whatever equipment they could to the back of the stage. Chairs and tables were flying, while bottles were being smashed and used as weapons. They bundled themselves into the back room behind the stage – they were in no doubt that the crowd would have gone for them as everything was out of control.

The band stayed hidden but chaos lasted for ages. Then came barking dogs and three blows of a whistle to signal the arrival of the police. Everyone stayed silent and still, figuring the best thing to do was to keep out of the way. Finally, some fifteen minutes later, it was completely silent and a policeman opened the door, telling them that they were safe to come out. The club was empty, but there was nothing left of it. Everything was smashed to smithereens. There wasn't a chair or table still standing, the bar had been decimated and there was blood everywhere. It was like a war zone. The episode traumatized the group, taking some of the joy and innocence away from their adventures on the road. The tour had allowed them to exist in a bubble but this was a big reality check and it let the world in, forcing Ted to be realistic about what was going on out there and at home. Deep down he knew that he couldn't keep running away for ever. The show continued travelling around the country until December 1974, when the gang went their separate ways.

Ted and Barry didn't keep in touch, but years later, when Ted's video went viral, Barry watched it online and knew immediately who it was:

'When I first saw that "Quando" video on Facebook, I knew it was Ted. He's still the same as he was then. Believe me, he's still got it. You know you get older and you may not look the same, but he's still the guy I knew back then. He was a good guy. I couldn't fault him and he always looked out for everyone, making sure they were alright, you know. He'd never make a fuss before a show. He'd pop on his suit, wait for the opening, walk on and do his thing.'

Once the tour was over, Ted returned to Wednesbury for a few weeks to spend some proper time at home. It was the first time he had truly dealt with Maurice's death – there was no escaping his absence, it was everywhere he looked. His siblings had made the initial adjustment but it was extremely raw for Ted and hard to process while still staying upbeat for Hilda, who loved having her eldest back home.

But before Ted had a chance to settle back into Wednesbury life, his talent for entertaining was about to take him somewhere, and to someone, he could never have anticipated. Butlin's had been so impressed with his ability to get on with everyone and all his ideas about how to breathe new life into the shows that, so the story goes, Billy Butlin's wife herself asked him personally to go to the Metropole Hotel in Blackpool to help their entertainment team. Before he knew it, Ted was off again, the promise of the bright lights luring him away from home – this time on a bus to Lancashire. As he prepared to say goodbye to the family again, he knew they were all wondering when he would stop gallivanting and start putting down roots. If he was honest, as he was approaching 40, he was starting to wonder that himself.

★★★

As soon as he arrived, Ted set about the job in hand. Even the building he would be working in was an institution in its own right. The Butlin's Metropole was a big red-brick hotel at the northern end of Blackpool promenade, just past the war memorial. It might be a bit of a faded treasure now but back then, in the mid-Seventies, it was the place to be. It seemed obvious to Ted that if the venue wasn't packing in the punters, then it had a lot to do with the quality of the acts they were putting on. The first thing Ted set about doing was scouting around all the clubs and pubs in Blackpool for the best talent. He would make notes and then go back to choose the best ones to appear at the Metropole. It didn't take long for the old hotel to become exactly the kind of place that Butlin's had been so desperate for.

There was now a buzz about the venue – it was the perfect place for a getaway. Soon news travelled to the other end of the country, reaching London and the ears of Linda Carter, a 29-year-old secretary from Blackburn. Linda had visited Blackpool hundreds of times over the years, but with her brother George away, she wanted to treat her parents to a New Year break. The Blackpool Metropole sounded ideal. She had no idea how much that holiday would change her world.

Linda Carter loved life. She had moved to London from Blackburn in 1971 when she was about 27 and was social, outgoing and fun. She'd rented a flat in St John's Wood and was earning a more-than-good wage working as a PA in Mayfair. But she never took work too seriously – to Linda it was just a chance to show off what she was wearing. She was devoted to fashion and the epitome of Seventies style – blonde bob, hotpants, big nails. Lunchtimes would be spent wandering around the shops – BIBA, Ossie Clark, Quorum and French Connection (back when it was just a boutique on the King's Road) – before strutting back to the office with her shopping, always late and without a care in the world. She loved London – it was an exciting place to be, and she felt anything was possible. Although she had a few flings and dates, nothing seemed to last and she wasn't bothered about settling down (much to her mother's concern). But it did mean she had something in common with the man she was about to meet.

That Christmas Linda took a break from London and went back to Blackburn to spend it with her mum and dad – George and Ellen Carter, two mill workers. They had just moved from a two-up, two-down terraced house in Bastwell to a semi-detached house with a front and back garden at the top of Little Harwood, bought after George had won some money on the pools.

George was a quiet yet confident man, and Blackburn born and bred. He was tall, smart and had been incredibly good-looking in his youth, while Ellen was a small, kind and honest woman with dyed red permed hair, but who wouldn't think twice about telling someone where to go if she felt they'd done her wrong. She was no battleaxe, but if anyone crossed her or her family, she would come down on them like a ton of bricks. Everyone knew her down in Little Harwood, her childhood home, where she'd spend hours mee-mawing to the other women in the shops, wearing Rainmates, pulling shopping trolleys and making sure she had the latest bargains. In many ways Linda's parents were very similar to Maurice and Hilda. It seemed ironic then, with such traditional role models who were very much in favour of marriage, that neither Linda nor Ted was in any hurry to find 'the one'.

On 29 December 1974, the Carters arrived at the Metropole Hotel. Ted McDermott opened the doors as they entered, immediately locking eyes with Linda: the attraction was instant. 'As soon as I saw her, I knew she was the one,' Ted used to say. 'I went straight to the other Redcoats and said, "If anyone talks to or touches that blonde, I'll break their legs. She's mine."' He had spent the last few years putting his romantic feelings on the backburner – women came and went but no one had captured his heart and mind for years – until now. It would be true to say that he loved Linda Carter from the moment he laid eyes on her – and that kind of attraction cannot be ignored.

That first afternoon they saw one another, Ted asked Linda for a game of table tennis. 'No, let's go for a walk instead,' said Linda and they spent the afternoon walking along a blustery Blackpool prom with Ted instantly charming her with his stories and jokes.

On New Year's Eve, Ted had organized a fancy dress competition in the main hotel ballroom. By this time Linda and her family had got to know a group of other people staying there, including a tall, thin guy, who was also holidaying with his family. He clearly had a bit of a crush on Linda because he followed her around and they always seemed to be together. Ted would watch from afar, not liking it one bit. He couldn't work out what was going on between them and drove himself mad with ideas about how he could get this guy out of the picture, clearing the way for himself. This was all made worse by the fact that Linda and the thin guy arrived at the New Year's Eve fancy dress party as a couple – the guy dressed as a Red Indian, who entered the room dragging Linda, who was dressed as a squaw, across the dance floor. It was an extravagant entrance and they won the competition.

For years afterwards Ted would say that he fixed the win, just to have a reason to talk to Linda, but she would insist they won fair and square because they were the best dressed in the competition.

Later that night, Linda went up to her room and changed out of her costume into something more glamorous, rejoining the crowd in the ballroom. As she came through the double doors, her eyes hit the stage in front of her. Everyone had gathered round it, watching a handsome guy singing onstage. She pushed her way through to get a better look at what was going on and found herself staring up at Ted singing.

'I remember him looking into my eyes as he sang, *We are in love again my heart and I.* My own heart melted and that was that.'

Solamente Una Vez

As the clocks struck midnight on 1 January 1975, Ted McDermott finally won over Linda Carter. To mark the occasion the couple decided to go paddling in the Blackpool sea. Over the years, neither one of them would give any detail about what went on out there, but one thing was certain: it was freezing.

The rest of Linda's stay passed in a romantic blur and she spent every possible moment with Ted, chatting and laughing as they walked around Blackpool – meaning he didn't get much work done and she didn't see a lot of her family. They were joined at the hip and completely smitten with each other. 'Ted was very much a romantic flatterer,' Linda says. 'He would always be telling me how lovely I was.'

But reality struck as the Christmas decorations came down and the guests started to go back home. Linda and Ted exchanged addresses and promises of visits and calls, but who knew what would happen? She returned to Blackburn with her parents for a few days before heading back to London – after all, they hadn't seen that much of her over the holiday period.

Linda was at her mum and dad's making the most of the final time she had left away from work when suddenly there was a knock at the door. She got up to see who was there, only to be confronted by a grinning Ted. She couldn't believe he was standing right there on her doorstep, only a few days after she had last seen him. It was a shock but it gently endeared Ted to her.

They spent the next day together and then decided to get the bus back down south, with Ted getting off at the Midlands to stay with his family and Linda continuing down to London. After another intense goodbye, they agreed that Linda would come and visit him at one of his gigs around the country, though no firm date was made; Ted didn't know where he was from one week to the next and had to be willing to go wherever the money and the jobs were.

The Butlin's tour was reassembled after Christmas and New Year, and Ted continued to be a major part of it, again travelling in that caravan with Dave Thomas. As Dave was putting Ted up, Ted would end up doing the cooking most nights, rustling up something quick and easy with whatever they had in the cupboards. It was a skill he had learned from an early age from Hilda – Ted would often cook for his younger siblings whenever his parents were out.

Being on the road meant he had lots to distract him from not seeing Linda, and equally, she loved her life in London. But Ted's nomadic lifestyle also meant that, inevitably, she ended up doing most of the travelling to see him. She would regularly spend hours on trains and buses, getting soaked to the skin in the north-east and stomping through sleet and snow in Scotland to get to whichever venue he was working in. Like Ted, she liked to make an impression and would always make sure she was wearing her best winter clothes when she arrived, which certainly turned a few heads. It also had the same effect on Ted, who loved the fact that she was there just to see him.

Although he wasn't the one making the long journey, Ted would make sure that everything was perfect for Linda's arrival. In fact, he made so much fuss about how the caravan looked that he drove Dave mad. Ted would clean the place obsessively until it was spotless before Linda arrived, and even when she was there he'd dust down the seats before she went to sit down. 'He was incredibly fussy,' Linda says. 'Everything would be polished to within an inch of its life. The place was spotless – I didn't think at that time I'd be hoovering up around him like I do now.' They were carefree times – travelling around from town to town with Dave driving, Ted sitting in the passenger seat and Linda in the back, with Dave's caravan attached to the rear of the car. All three of them would joke and sing their way through the long journeys. It was a joy for Linda and a world away from her nine-to-five life in London. There was a real sense of freedom and that anything was possible; she could see why Ted found it so seductive.

Things fell into a natural pattern for Ted and Linda and they were serious from the beginning and very much a part of each other's lives, even if Ted being on the road made communication tricky. Linda met Hilda and the rest of Ted's relatives at the first opportunity. In truth, as far as Hilda was concerned, it was an enormous relief that he seemed to have found someone so kind and capable to settle down with.

By Easter 1975, Linda would regularly spend all of her weekends travelling from London to see Ted. 'I was absolutely cracked,' she remembers. 'I used to turn up in my big coat and big hat in all sorts of weather. We stayed everywhere – B&Bs, old hotels – basically, anywhere that catered for travelling entertainers.' It was a rough-and-ready existence but Ted would make sure he kept the romance alive. During the Easter weekend he was tidying the caravan and came across a woollen hat of Linda's. As a surprise, he decided to spend the whole afternoon making paper flowers from serviettes he'd been given at the club. He then stuck each flower into the hat, turning it into an Easter bonnet that she would wear that night to the pub for a laugh.

Ted courted Linda as if his life depended on it, but things took on a whole new complexion at the end of April 1975, when Linda found out she was pregnant after visiting the doctor in London. She wasn't shocked by the news and knew immediately she would keep the baby

– even when she was offered an abortion as an unmarried woman. Linda had no idea how Ted would react – they hadn't been together that long and he was very much a free spirit who loved seeing where the wind took him. That kind of life, without stability or routine, was the opposite of what a baby needed – Linda didn't know if Ted could give her what she and her child needed, or even if he wanted to be involved. The knowledge that she was keeping her baby, no matter what Ted said, made telling him a lot easier than it might have been. Preparing herself to sit him down to deliver such life-changing news did bring into sharp focus exactly how much they didn't know about each other.

So, the next weekend she was scheduled to see him, Linda let Ted pick her up from the station and, once they were back at the caravan, she took his hand: 'You're going to be a dad.' There was silence.

Ted took in the news and then finally said:

'We should get married.'

Linda was surprised at how calm he was. In fact, everyone seemed laid-back, including Linda's parents. It wasn't the ideal way round but Hilda was over the moon when she heard the news that Ted was going to be a father. She would tell anyone who would listen how beautiful Linda was and, privately, she knew a baby meant Ted would have to put down roots and stop acting like a teenager on the cusp of 'making it big'.

The pregnancy news wasn't the life-altering bombshell Linda thought it might be. In fact, by the summer, life had quickly returned to its usual routine – Ted was back at Butlin's and she was back to the office, travelling up to see Ted whenever she could. Keen not to be limited by the pregnancy, Linda carried on as normal, even taking off to Canada for a three-week holiday. It was a modern arrangement and one that suited them both – Linda didn't want the world from Ted and he was relieved not to be suffocated by it all.

But even though the parents-to-be were happy to carry on as usual, there were practicalities to address and, as is often the way, their own parents wished to impress upon them their responsibilities. The biggest issue was deciding where the baby would be raised. Linda had planned to stay in London and rent a bigger flat so that Ted could live with her. Her parents weren't keen on that idea, as she would be far away from family support and on her own with a newborn while Ted was out and about travelling to find work. It just didn't seem practical and they worried that Linda didn't understand the pressure a new baby would bring and how much life would change. Eventually, and after much discussion, Linda's mum managed to persuade her to leave London and move back to Blackburn so that she could help with the baby. In fact, the most sensible thing was for Linda to move back home and take the back bedroom for her, Ted and the new baby.

Although it wasn't ideal, Linda knew deep down that it was the right solution and that she would need all the help she could get. But even she had no idea just how much that family support would be needed, especially as the autumn progressed and she slowly stopped hearing from Ted. There was no specific event that caused the fracture, more that they simply stopped talking to each other as much as they had at the beginning of their relationship. Ted kept odd hours because of his performances and could rarely get to a telephone, and Linda stopped being able to make the long journey to see him due to her condition. Even all these years later all Linda will say is: 'We just drifted away from each other – I don't know what happened – we just didn't seem to contact each other that much. It's not like today when you could just pick up a phone or send a text. People lost contact easily.' Both sets of parents soon learned that it was better not to ask too many questions, which was something that Hilda found difficult to manage given that Ted was due to move back home after the summer once the Butlin's season was over.

When Ted did come home with his suitcases full of laundry, exhausted and a little manic after months of performing every night, it was as if he was in denial and Linda hadn't happened. He set about finding work in factories and wherever else he could; at first Hilda assumed he was saving for the baby's arrival, but it was hard to tell as he simply didn't mention the situation. Never one to keep her opinions to herself, Hilda managed three whole days before being unable to contain her curiosity any more. As Ted made them both a cup of tea one morning, she turned to him and blurted out:

'What's happening with you and this girl having your baby? What yam playing at?'

Ted could feel Hilda's eyes burning into his back as she waited for him to answer. She continued: 'Your dad would be turning in his grave – we didn't bring you up to ignore your responsibilities.'

Finally, the couple did eventually make contact and a visit was arranged as the baby's due date drew nearer.

They agreed to meet at Hilda's. Linda was anxious – she hadn't seen Ted for months, she felt tired, emotional and full of uncertainty. As she sat on the train to Wednesbury, she was happy that she would soon see Ted again. She arrived at 18 Kent Road, opened the gate and knocked on the door. But it wasn't Ted who answered, it was Ted's sister, Marilyn, who offered her a cup of tea. It soon became clear that he wasn't there at all. Hilda fussed around and did all she could to hide the fact that she didn't know Linda was coming and she had no idea where Ted was – the one thing she did know was that she wanted to swing for him.

A couple of hours of small talk later, Ted suddenly burst through the door and the couple were reunited. As ever, Ted fussed around Linda, taking her to the local pub where he introduced her to his old friend Norman Deeley. Hilda was so concerned with how things might turn out because of Ted's behaviour that she even offered to raise the baby herself once it was born, despite her grief over Maurice and her failing health. It was the desperate act of a woman terrified she would be cut out of her grandchild's life.

But she needn't have worried. Linda had already vowed never to stop Ted being a father to their child. In fact, she took to sending tapes down to him so that he knew how the pregnancy was progressing and how she was getting on. 'I remember when those tapes used to arrive,' says Karen, one of Ted's younger sisters. 'We'd often sit around listening to them – but then there'd always be one that he'd take upstairs and listen to on his own.'

Christmas 1975. Ted's brother Fred was now a driver for sales reps around the country.

'You ever get up around Blackburn way?' asked Ted. 'That girlfriend of mine is having a nipper and I could do with popping up.'

'You tell me when it is, our Big, so I can arrange things around it.'

'Well, it could be in the next day or so…'

★★★

At 12.40 p.m., just after Christmas on 29 December 1975, I was born and Linda and Ted became my mum and dad. My arrival changed everything as far as Hilda was concerned – she told Dad in no uncertain terms that he needed to step up. A few days later, Dad was driven to Blackburn by Uncle Fred. After a couple of hours driving up from Wednesbury, they finally arrived, pulling up outside a pub. The wind was howling, with big sheets of metal being blown around like pieces of cardboard.

'Look here, our kid. Tonight I'll sit in this pub and wait for you. At bang on 9.30, I'll be getting in the car and going home, and if yam not here by then, you're on your own,' said Fred.

Dad made his way to Bramley Meade maternity home in Whalley, near Blackburn, clutching a blue teddy bear, where he would meet his son, me, for the first time.

After Fred finished work, he sat in the pub waiting a good few hours for Dad to return, fully expecting he wouldn't arrive on time. Just as the clock on the wall turned to half-past nine, Dad burst through the doors. 'Her's had a little lad. You wanna see him, our Fred. He's a McDermott alright!'

'He walked in like he owned the bloody pub,' says Fred.

Despite the unorthodox circumstances, Dad was over the moon to be a father. 'You know he was so proud when he had a son,' says John. 'He was always proud of you, you know. He always said that if his boy wanted to do something, he'd want him to be able to do it. He didn't want anything to hold back his son.'

It makes my heart glow thinking how Dad felt about me, but it also makes me wonder whether I did turn out to make him as proud as he was right at that moment when I was born.

The next day, I was registered as Simon Edward Carter – no one expected my on/off parents to get married, so I was given Mum's maiden name and Dad's middle name. At least I was given what Mum *thought* was Dad's middle name – in another ridiculous reminder that the new parents really didn't know each other, it turned out that Dad's middle name was, in fact, Edmund.

My birth triggered something in Dad, just as Hilda had prayed it would, and the day after his visit to Bramley Meade, he wrote Mum a long letter, saying how much he loved her and wanted to spend the rest of his life with her, including the infamous words: 'If I could put you in my top pocket next to my heart I would.' Mum thought it sounded ridiculous and laughed as she showed it to Nan, who had been less than impressed with the way Dad had shrugged off his responsibilities. Mum expected that my nan would greet the letter with a healthy measure of cynicism and dismissiveness – after all, she didn't think Dad was capable of much. So imagine her surprise when Nan read the letter, folded it back into its envelope and turned, with tears in her eyes, to say: 'Linda, it's once in a lifetime you'll get a letter like that! He completely loves you.'

It wasn't the most romantic moment of Mum's life, but Mum and Dad decided to take their vows at Blackburn Register Office on 7 February 1976. Someone had finally achieved the impossible and made Dad settle down – he was 39 and Mum was 31.

No one is sure if the wedding gave Mum the security she needed – she was smart and knew that a wedding ring was no guarantee of anything. She also didn't want to be with him because he felt they should be – she made it perfectly clear that she was more than capable and willing to raise me alone. Mum was not duty bound to Dad or anyone else. She was realistic enough to know that Dad wouldn't ever be a millionaire – a joke she shared with her mum on the morning of the wedding – 'I probably won't be rich in money but at least I will be rich in love.'

Mum was bang on trend when it came to her wedding outfit, shunning the classic virginal white gown. Instead she wore a pale grey suit, pink top and her old brown school beret, which Grandad had been wearing a few days earlier to do some painting – if you looked closely it was still possible to see the paint flecks. She finished off the look with a fox fur draped around her neck – an idea she got after watching the wedding of the Earl of Lichfield on television – making her feel a million dollars. Dad was uncharacteristically restrained and wore a plain navy-blue suit. His best man was his brother, Malcolm, and Mum's maid of honour was her close friend, Edna, who had arranged to drive Mum and Dad to Blackburn Register Office on the day.

As with all good love stories, the big day itself was fraught, with Edna caught up in a suspected IRA bombing in Birmingham, meaning she and her husband David couldn't get to their car to drive up as planned. But a policeman took pity on them and they sped up the motorway, making it to Nan and Grandad's house to find Mum and Dad standing at the bus stop opposite, waiting for the number 14 to go into town.

In another break with convention, both the bride and groom's mothers stayed away: Hilda, due to illness and the fact it was so far for her to travel, and Nan because she was so appalled at the idea of me being at the ceremony. When asked why she was missing the most important day of her daughter's life, she snapped back: 'No way is this baby going to his own mother's wedding!'

Nan stood at the front-room window, clutching me and laughing to herself as she watched Edna and David bundle Mum and Dad in the back of their car and then speed off. She knew her headstrong daughter was resilient and determined to do things her own way – after all, she had even bought her own wedding ring (much to the dismay of Nan, who thought Dad probably 'had enough in his drawers to use as curtain rings'). Nan prayed Dad and Mum would be happy, but she couldn't shake the heavy feeling that there was a rocky road ahead. She had tried to come around to Dad and they did have a unique relationship, which mainly consisted of lots of bickering and bantering. Nan found the best way to communicate with her future son-in-law was to affectionately mock his ego. They could regularly be overheard trading insults when Dad came to stay in the run-up to the wedding and it got worse as the years progressed. Mum would roll her eyes as she walked into the front room to hear Nan shouting: 'Your head's so big that it would take two strong men to carry it on a platter', to which he would reply: 'Maybe so – but if I put my head in your mouth it would still rattle.' Later on, Dad would invite Nan along to any show he was doing, but then introduce her to the audience as a famous, one-legged clog dancer, which had everyone in stitches. Each was determined to outsmart the other and it was an endless competition as well as being an affectionate way for the two of them to draw the necessary battle lines and keep each other in check.

In keeping with the unconventional tone set by the couple, the wedding itself provided some unintentional humour – beginning with the best man being struck down with a laughing fit and chuckling throughout the ceremony from beginning to end. No one could understand why Malcolm found such a serious commitment so hilarious. But when asked what he was laughing at, he said: 'I just couldn't believe our Ted was getting married at last.' At the end of the ceremony, Edna turned to Linda and said: 'You've done it now, kid.' To which Linda replied: 'Well, I like to try everything once.'

The wedding party then all walked up to Tommy Balls to do a spot of bargain-hunting at the once-legendary Blackburn shoe shop. After that, they all caught the bus back to Little Harwood, where Nan had put on a buffet for everyone, followed by a meal at the Saxon Hotel. It might have been a small wedding, but it was perfect. 'To be honest I wasn't that bothered about getting married,' says Mum. 'It's just something we had to do. There were no grand speeches, no big cake, no dancing and no fuss, but we were there and we were married, and that was that.'

The low-key theme continued – there wasn't even a honeymoon. Mum and Dad just carried on with life as they knew it. On the Monday after the wedding, my name was changed from Simon Carter to Simon McDermott, Dad went back to work in Wednesbury, travelling up to Blackburn every few weeks or so to see us, while Mum and me stayed at Nan and Grandad's.

Mum and Dad would spend their free time going dancing at St Stephen's Club or one of the many other clubs in Blackburn. In the meantime, Dad had changed his stage name to Eddie Carter. Carter was both Hilda and Mum's maiden name and it seemed the perfect fit. In fact, everything felt like it had finally fallen into place for him and

Dad's family couldn't have agreed more. 'Linda Carter was the best thing that happened to him,' Fred would tell anyone who listened. 'She put him right financially and taught him how to look after his money. You can imagine what he was like – he was only interested in music. Me, Colin and the rest of the brothers had all settled down, got our own house, but he'd just want to go out and do his music. That was the only thing that mattered to him.'

Now he had a wife and a son that mattered just as much and this was Ted's chance to finally have his 'happy ever after'.

The Songaminute Man

By June 1976, Dad accepted he had to make a permanent move to Blackburn. It was a sobering moment and one that nearly broke Hilda's heart. Over the years she had lost her sons to their new wives and eventual children, and had been desperate for Dad to follow suit and settle down, but when the day arrived for him to leave, she was devastated. Dad packed up his things and set off for Little Harwood, where he would move in with his in-laws, much to the amusement of his brothers.

Finding work was obviously the priority and he set about looking for a job, finding one at Premier Construction – a factory that made prefabricated buildings, just five minutes across the dual carriageway from Nan and Grandad's house. The week before the factory had just installed a new wood machine.

'Have you used anything like this before?' the foreman asked Dad.

'No, but if you show me how to use it, I'll give it a go.'

No one had much hope that Dad would settle, but as with the wedding, he surprised everyone and ended up working at Premier as a wood machinist for the next seventeen years of his life. In hindsight, he probably hated it. He'd gone from being a single man, performing in shows most nights, to living with his wife's parents and working in a factory. He'd also gone from living in Wednesbury, where everyone knew him, to a town where no one had a clue who he was. It must have been a huge shock and, for someone like him, a blow to the ego. But no one would have have known as he just got on with what needed to be done.

Geoff Sutton worked with Dad at Premier: 'He was a great guy and a good grafter – he worked hard, you know, he never skived off. Ted worked in the machine shop and he'd always be singing – trying to learn the words to songs or something. I remember one work trip we all went to Aintree to the races, and at the end of the night, Ted got up and sang in the club.

'I also remember one other time, just after he'd first started, Linda came into the factory asking where he was. I pointed her over and next thing I knew she was hitting him over the head with her bag. She was going ballistic about something or other. We all kept out of it – he was in the doghouse that day!'

Dad quickly fell into the role of family man – illustrated best in July 1976, when the entire family went to a Pontins holiday camp in Southport. He entered the talent competition and won, winning a week's holiday and a plastic mock-gold trophy in the shape of a winged angel. The trophy still sits on the mantelpiece at home to this day: 'Pontins' Star Quest Winner 1976'.

With full-time work, being a husband and a new father, Dad let his singing slip. But Mum soon put a stop to that. She knew he loved singing, and besides, she'd fallen in love with a singer.

'When I met you, you said you were a singer. If you're not going to go singing, then you know where the door is!' she ranted at him during one of their many arguments.

So he started going out and taking bookings at the clubs in Blackburn. One of the first places he went to was St Stephen's Club, just down the road from his in-laws' house in Little Harwood. St Stephen's was a traditional northern club: downstairs was the main room with a small stage, with a smaller snooker room off the side;

upstairs was another function room with a slightly bigger stage. On the wall there was a picture of the Queen. In the summer, the green outside was packed with all the members playing bowls. These days though, the club has gone – changes in the local population mean that there's no longer the demand for it.

Rose Boothman, a regular at the club, remembers the first time she met Dad: 'I remember when he first came to the club,' she says. 'He was on his own and got talking to my husband, Jimmy. After a while Jim said, "Come and sit with us, lad, yer a good un," so he did.' That night St Stephen's was having a 'free and easy' night – meaning that anyone could get up and sing if they wanted.

'Go on up and have a go, lad,' Jimmy told Dad.

So Dad got up and he knocked them all out. 'The way he hit those top notes,' says Rose. 'The roof lifted. He was BRILLIANT.'

When Dad sat back down with the group, Jimmy turned to him and said: 'You should think about doing the clubs, lad.'

'I've already done them down the Midlands,' said Dad, and began to tell Jimmy, who was one of the compères as well as being vice-president of the club, all about his time at Butlin's and where he met Mum.

From then on, Jimmy and Dad became good friends – often Jimmy and Rose would have a party back at their house in Bastwell with some of the regulars, including Mum and Dad, after the club had shut. The couples were friends right up until Jimmy's death and the onset of Dad's dementia, but even then, the illness couldn't quite rob Dad of all his memories: 'When Jimmy died, Ted used to walk past our house every morning and touch that hedge there,' says Rose. 'I'd watch him from upstairs. Every morning without fail, he'd walk past, touch the hedge and shout, "Morning, Jimmy", and walk off. Every morning he'd do it. Jimmy was always cutting that hedge and they'd always be talking when he passed. It just became this thing that he did after Jimmy died. Every morning.'

Blackburn in the mid-1970s was a hotspot. There were clubs all across town, often featuring live entertainment most nights of the week. It's crazy to think that most of Blackburn's pubs and clubs have now closed, either having been demolished, becoming derelict or religious education centres. There is very little left of the club scene it once was, but back then it was thriving and Dad made sure he was at the heart of it. Most weekends Mum and Dad would go out, leaving me at Nan's, and it was almost as though they were courting again. They would go to the clubs and Dad would often end the night by getting up and singing – especially if it was an open-mic night. He soon found that everyone locally knew who he was and looked forward to hearing his voice.

Ernie Riding was one of the regular piano players at St Stephen's Club at the time – a tall guy with a broad Lancashire accent and black hair. When I was a kid he seemed like the typical showman – smart suits and buckets of confidence. He was a self-taught pianist and could play any song by ear. Combined with Dad's musical knowledge they would often have a great flow together, mashing up different songs and styles, which was impressive to watch.

It was often at these nights at St Stephen's that Dad showcased his medleys – a non-stop mix of as many songs as they could sing in the time available. By the end of the set, Dad and Ernie would be racing through music hall classics: Baby Face, If You Knew Susie, California Here I Come, to name but a few. The whole crowd would be on their feet, applauding and shouting for more. By now, he had begun to get a bit of a name for himself, not just because of this but also due to his vast knowledge of songs spanning generations: there was nothing he couldn't sing. One night, just before his usual set, the compère at the club (who happened to be Jimmy Boothman) accidentally gave him a new name as he announced him to the crowd:

'Here he is, Eddie Carter – The Songaminute Man.'

That was it – the name stuck, and from then on it was how Dad was known throughout Blackburn.

'You know, he could sing any style,' says Ernie. 'Those medleys were a lot of fun. He made you work and sometimes they'd go on for ages. I can remember being covered in sweat, but it was a lot of fun. Then he'd also go on to do the serious songs. They were quality. I remember him when he first came in. He wanted to do a spot, it was a free and easy. I knew the moment he started singing he was quality. From then on we gelled.'

Ernie had a small group that he would also do private gigs with and over the next twenty or so years Dad would always sing with him. 'If there were any special jobs on, I'd always ask Eddie,' he says. 'You dad was never a big head – but he always had talent. I'm not just saying it, but he was one of a kind. He was either singing or joking and what he didn't know about music wasn't worth knowing. He could go right back to the Twenties and sing Al Bowlly stuff. He was quite unique – I was always proud to play with him.'

But it was clear that Dad didn't try and hide his more artistic temperament from Ernie. 'You know, if he didn't like a musician he would walk off. I've seen him walk off the stage if he didn't like the pianist. But then again I've done the same with singers,' says Ernie. The two men formed a close friendship that was pivotal in helping Dad settle down in Blackburn – he was miles away from his brothers and sisters, so it was a huge relief to Mum when he and Ernie clicked so early on. Having music in common was a huge bonus and she was happy he was part of a circle he could socialize with.

As ever in small towns, word started to spread, and through Ernie, Dad soon became known to Alf Wright – who himself was known as Blackburn's Mr Music. He was a plumber by trade, who started to organize shows at Blackburn's King George's Hall. 'He wasn't a musician or singer,' says Ernie, 'but he just loved music and wanted to put on these shows. It was all the stuff from mine and Ted's era.'

For years afterwards, Dad would always have the occasional gig at King George's as part of Alf Wright's Music Hall – either singing, compèring or both. One thing that stood out was his confidence and stage presence – it became the talk of Blackburn and soon he had pockets full of booking requests and gigs lined up months in advance. To celebrate this Mum went out and bought him an expensive dress shirt for his shows. But when he found out, Dad went ballistic because she'd spent the extra money on it. 'Eddie, if you take £1 from every booking you got on Sunday, that will pay for the price of the shirt two times,' she yelled.

This small fall-out characterized a tricky time for the newly-weds and they argued a lot as they adjusted to making a life together. Here were two people who had previously been committed to the single life and suddenly they had a baby, were living with a set of parents and struggling to make ends meet. Mum missed the buzz of London and he missed the freedom of being on the road – maintaining their new life was putting a lot of pressure on them both. For Mum, one of the main problems was that when Dad did a big show, he wouldn't want to go into work the next day. This caused a lot of resentment, both from Mum and my ever-observant nan, who watched Dad closely for signs he wasn't looking after her daughter. They didn't understand the performer's mentality – how much it took out of Dad to be up on that stage all night. They were much more familiar with a nine-to-five routine and the stability it brought. To them not going to work was just lazy, but for Dad, he needed time to recover.

It all came to a head after a few weeks when, after one late night gig, Dad refused to get out of the bed the next morning to help with me or go to work. Mum was exasperated and stomped down to the kitchen, complaining to my nan that her husband was useless. 'That's it,' muttered Nan, watching her tired and stressed daughter juggle everything as her husband snored in bed. She went to the cupboard under the stairs and pulled out the hoover, marched up to Mum and Dad's bedroom, switched it on, and left it running. Dad snapped. He got up, packed his bag and went to live at the YMCA. It was a huge drama – but Nan wasn't at all repentant. Her own husband wasn't lazy and her daughter wasn't going to put up with that and she told Dad as much.

This exile didn't last long though, and my parents were soon back together, but staying with the in-laws indefinitely wasn't an option. After getting gazumped on a small cottage, they put their names down for a council house. And a few weeks later, they moved into Number 2 Windermere Close, Daisyfield, in July 1977. It was a small end-of-terrace 1960s build, with a tiny garden at the front and the back. They made it their own, furnishing it with things they picked up from junk shops or jumble sales.

By summer 1977, Mum and Dad decided to book their first summer holiday alone and decided to go to the tiny Cornish seaside town of Bude. They were so excited; Mum set about buying new clothes and planning all the things they would do and where they would eat. But this happy time turned to heartbreak for Dad when his beloved mother died on what would have been her sixtieth birthday. Although her health had rapidly declined since the death of her husband Maurice, no one expected her to go so soon. She had been getting to grips with her diabetes, which had the worrying side effect of causing her to faint or lose her balance. It was one final fall at home from a diabetic coma that led to her being taken to hospital and dying there, quickly and unexpectedly. It was a crushing blow for her family, who were still adjusting to life without Maurice. Everyone was in shock and it would take many years for Dad to come to terms with this loss.

Despite being devastated, Dad still went to work the next day. Mum called them up to explain what had happened and asked them to keep an eye on him. 'He didn't want people to see that he was upset half the time,' she said. When Dad returned back to Kent Road for the funeral, he just opened the door and went straight upstairs. 'That was his thing when he was upset – he would just walk straight upstairs and not talk to anyone,' says my Auntie Karen. Just before the funeral, Dad spent time with Hilda's body at the funeral home and sat with her for hours, his conversation committed to history and the depths of his now-muddled mind. His mother had been his world and now he was living in a new town, with a new wife and a new baby. It was a lot for him to process and perhaps he never fully did.

Hilda was buried with her beloved Maurice, leaving her children to come to terms with the fact that such a big force was gone for ever. She had been the centre of the family, but now she wasn't there. And even though each of them had their own households, becoming an orphan at any age is life-changing: suddenly there is no one around who knew you from the very start. Dad dealt with it by silently getting on with things, but it took its toll on his marriage and saw the start of an exhausting and destructive pattern of rowing, splitting up and making up – a cycle that can eat away at the foundations of even the strongest relationship.

Perhaps Hilda's death triggered a fear of loss in Dad, perhaps he was just a jealous person, but either way, he became extremely possessive of Mum and didn't care who saw it.

This was most obvious during their first Christmas together after Hilda's death, when they spent Boxing Day with Mum's friends Edna and David. The two women were still close after the wedding when Edna had been Mum's maid of honour and it sounded like a fun idea to spend some of the holidays with her and her husband. The pair had a fancy-dress box and Edna's brother, Brian, and Mum dressed up and acted out a comedy sketch. Dad didn't like this. As

Mum and Brian came waltzing down the stairs all dressed up, Dad went ballistic, storming out of the house and walking all the way back home – which was over five miles away. It was embarrassing for Mum that her friends saw that side to him and it became clear that it wasn't just something you could put down to the fact he was an emotional or highly strung artist. Other times, when Mum went out alone with her friends, Dad would lock her out of the house in a fit of jealousy, leaving her to walk up to Nan and Grandad's house, where she would stay the night.

But Mum was no doormat and could only be pushed so far. One morning, she had decided to get up early and make a full breakfast of bacon and eggs to set Dad up for the day, just the way Hilda used to before he went off to work. She thought maybe some home comforts would help him come to terms with things and remind him of good times even though he was sad. Her loving gesture backfired spectacularly as it became clear that Dad wasn't in the mood for niceties.

'I don't want this,' he said, pushing his breakfast away. 'I like my eggs runny.'

But he couldn't have been sitting in a worse position. Right behind him was a china pot, in the shape of a chicken, where they kept all the eggs. Mum turned around, picked up an egg and smashed it right on the top of his head.

'Is this runny enough for you?' she shouted, storming through the door and making a run for it. Dad saw the funny side, chasing after her down the road and grabbing her with both hands. 'I love you, Linda McDermott,' he declared, right there in the road, with the neighbours getting a good look. They must have thought they were crazy.

But by mid-1978 the bickering had reached new levels and Mum walked out on Dad. 'Looking back, I can't even remember what we argued about half the time,' she says. 'I think we were both very argumentative and always wanted our own way. They were silly arguments but they would turn into World War Three. We were both to blame.'

Mum and I moved back to Nan's house – this time she was serious about splitting up for good. She had tried to be understanding after Hilda's death, but that jealous and argumentative streak in Dad just got worse and their relationship had become a battleground. So she left, taking me with her.

Jambalaya

On the surface, it all seemed very civilized – they split their money and Mum bought her own house, 138 Cedar Street, near Bastwell in Blackburn. It was a mid-terrace house and tiny, but it was hers and she loved it. The street was a typical red-bricked Lancashire terraced street – everyone knew each other and I spent my early years playing out with other kids from the street and building important friendships.

There was Jason a few doors down, who was to become my best friend at the time; Ellen, who lived on Bastwell Road; Kathryn and her brother, Michael, were across the street; Louise, with her broken blue NHS glasses and a patch over one eye, lived further down opposite the laundrette with her younger brother, Brett; John, the redhead of the group, who lived up Logwood Street; and Shirley McKenna, who lived on the corner opposite. We all hung out together, often making our way down to Jim's Shop to buy 5p Lucky Bags or playing out in the backstreets. Next door to us lived Bloody Mary – an old woman who would sit in her porch all day, moaning about 'bloody this' and 'bloody that'. On the other side was a tiny hairdresser's, with a small yapping terrier called Scooby Doo that never stopped barking. Next to her was Ida, who was forever sweeping the street. And next to her was Big John, with his two pet poodles, Pepsi and Shirlie.

Mrs Goodrich lived further down the street. She was an old lady who lived alone and who was forever telling us off. Of course I didn't know these people when we first moved in, but they became like family until I was 8 years old. Everyone knew each other. We got told off, we were given sweets, we'd go into each other's houses and dare each other to see how far we could walk down the walls in the back alley or play in the derelict garages behind Louise's house. I used to have a little yellow plastic car that you could sit on and drive when I was very young, but by the time I was about 7, we took it from the house, up the top of Holly Street, and would fly down on it to the bottom of the hill, missing cars driving across the street by inches. It was a wonder we didn't get killed. When my dad saw this, he flew out the house and gave me a good hiding. I never did that again.

Mum and Dad's separation wasn't to last. After she left, Dad took a long hard look at himself. He wanted Mum and me back but he knew things had to change. He also knew that Hilda would have been disappointed at the split, telling him to sort himself out – this wasn't a game and he needed to step up. Everyone else might celebrate and revere him, letting him get away with murder because of his voice – but his wife didn't.

Dad missed Mum like crazy, and he set out to win her back, waiting for her every night after work. She initially refused but was eventually worn down and charmed by Dad's persistence – he would be there as she finished work every night, waiting with a little gift and a smile.

'It drove me round the bend at first,' says Mum. 'I was dead set about moving on, but he managed to win me round. I remember that day. I'd come home from work and gone to my mum's to pick you up when I saw him standing at the top of the road, all dressed up, waiting for me. It was like a scene out of *Wuthering Heights* or something. I don't know what happened. Something just clicked and we ran to one another and started kissing. I must have been mad.'

As both my parents went back to work straight after I was born, it was my nan and grandad who looked after me during the day. Dad would pick me up at 4.15 on the dot. He'd knock off at 4 p.m. and it would take exactly 15 minutes for him to walk down from his workplace, Premier. I can still hear it now – the gate of Nan and Grandad's front garden opening and then Dad whistling or singing as he came up the path.

Dad was a natural with kids – he was surrounded by them growing up and his time at Butlin's further cemented that skill. Some parents read storybooks to their kids, but he wasn't like that – his stories were all in his head and he'd just recite them on the spot, often making them far more elaborate as he acted them out. Whenever we'd walk to John's Cut Price – the corner shop – together to pick up his cigarettes, he'd share these tales with me. For years I told everyone that my parents met when my dad was walking along Blackpool prom and saw an old pile of rags in the gutter. He heard a little voice shouting 'Help me! Help me!' and, after looking around for ages, Dad eventually saw a little fairy stuck underneath the pile of rags. He picked her up and put her in his top pocket, and she became my mum. Then there was the story of how the goldfish got its name. Again, this involved a fairy, but this time trapped in a bubble in a stream. All the other fishes ignored it, until eventually the ugliest, dirtiest fish in the stream swam along and popped the bubble, freeing the fairy. To thank him, the fairy turned him into a golden fish, but with a small black spot near its eye, to remind the other fairies and fish that he was the one who saved her. 'If you see a goldfish with a black spot, Sime, that's the one that saved the fairy!' he'd say and then we'd spend hours looking in the fishtanks at Animal Magic on Blackburn Market to see if we could spot it. At night time when we'd walk to the chip shop, we'd look up to the stars and he would tell me how each star was one of my ancestors looking down on me – the brightest, of course, were his parents, Hilda and Maurice.

At bedtime, he would prepare me for sleep with one of his epic fables, filled with fairies and farmyard animals, all concocted on the spot. I'd cling to every word, not wanting it to end. Then, as I began to nod off, he'd tuck me in and ruffle my hair. 'Remember – you're the best!' he would say, before switching off the light.

As a young child, I was obsessed by the story of *The Three Billy Goats Gruff* and convinced that they lived in Roe Lee Park, just down the road. When we all went there, we would go down to the small stream and act out the plot. Dad would hide under the bridge pretending to be a troll, while Mum and I would pretend to be goats crossing. Every so often he would jump out from under the bridge, scaring the life out of us. And I was convinced he could kick a football up through the sky. 'Do it again, Dad, do it again!' I'd shout as I watched this tiny ball go high up into the heavens, thinking that it would go so far that it would never come back. To me, he was amazing – although he wouldn't think twice about giving me a clip round the ear if I did anything wrong.

However, there was still a lot of drama in my parents' relationship. As well as collecting me, it was Dad's job to drop me off at Nan and Grandad's each morning. He left the house at 7.15 on the dot as his shift started at 7.30. We raced up Laburnum Road, past derelict factories, and I'd be dropped off to start the day with a cupful of raisins and a glass of Vimto.

It was during one of these mornings that I remember just about getting to the end of Cedar Street near St James Road with my dad, when I heard this almighty scream: it was Mum. 'Here! Here's your clothes!' and then all Dad's clothes were thrown from the front door into the middle of the street. Then the door banged shut.

As a child I was terrified. Dad turned around and we both walked back towards the house.

Just as we got to the door, it swung open again. This time it was all Dad's records.

'And you can take your records too!'

I knew that wasn't a good sign.

Mum and Dad always had an explosive and passionate relationship, punctuated by huge rows and then making up. Both stubborn and independent, they were also bound together. They loved each other and, old-fashioned as it might seem, it was very much 'for better or worse'.

Dad had been a caring child and that compassion for others continued into his adult years and the workplace. Dad showed this side to his boss at Premier. When he got to work one day, a group of blokes were stood around in the canteen. 'Here, Ted, Astley's upstairs, crying at his desk,' one of them said. Astley was the boss; he'd built up the company along with his partner from scratch. Dad went upstairs to the offices and sure enough found Astley sat in his office with his head in his hands, crying his eyes out. Dad walked straight in. 'Right, what's going on with you?' he asked.

The story goes that the company was in trouble and that, combined with the fact a number of the guys had decided to go on strike, had pushed Astley over the edge.

'Yam being daft. Everyone here wants to support you. You're a good boss and we all want the work. Listen, I'll go down there and tell them what's going on. None of this matters. What matters is that you're OK and you stop cracking up. And then afterwards, me and you are going to the races,' Dad apparently told him.

That afternoon Dad and Astley went to the races, with Astley driving them in his car. 'He hadn't a clue what he was doing, but the first bet he put on, he bloody won two hundred quid!' Dad told people at the time. 'He was a good boss, he just let things get on top of him. He had a lot of worries.' This was typical of Dad – he could feel the pain of others, which is perhaps why he felt his own emotions so keenly, something Iris had been so very aware of when they dated.

Dad knew everyone on Cedar Street. He was forever chatting and joking with Mrs Goodrich (the old lady who was forever telling us off) and Bloody Mary (the battleaxe next door). 'It was because he thought they were lonely,' Mum would say. 'He'd always go out of his way to talk to anyone if he thought they were lonely – he never liked to see people being on their own.'

Mrs Goodrich was divorced and was always stood in her front porch telling us off. 'Looking back, I think she probably had depression or something,' Mum says. 'But your dad would always make the time to say hello or talk to her for ages each time we passed. She was a nice lady – she was just fed up with you kids playing outside her house all day.'

I still remember Bloody Mary sat in her front porch – curlers in her hair, floral pinny, arms folded over her baby-pink cardigan and a face like a Rottweiler – watching our every move. I was scared of her because I knew if she saw me doing anything (walking on someone's back wall, for example), my dad would know about it straight away. Then I'd get a clip round the ear and be dragged round to hers to apologize. Years later, I bumped into her in Blackburn Market and she was the nicest old lady you could ever meet.

As an only child with no brothers or sisters, I was desperate to have a pet, but nothing really went to plan initially. First there was Monty the black cat – but it got run over by the bus after just a few months. Grandad had to scoop it up from the road with a shovel. Next I was given a rabbit – although that didn't last long either. I excitedly showed it to the dog next door, leading to it having a heart attack and dying in my arms, its eyes wide open in fright. Later that day, Dad took me up to the field behind the factory on Laburnum Road, dug a grave and buried it there, while I said the Lord's Prayer on repeat.

Dad soon began building a small extension at the back of the house – which I convinced myself was going to be a stable for a horse.

I sat on the backyard wall with the rest of the kids from the street, showing them where it would be. You can imagine my devastation when I was told it was going to be nothing more than a lean-to on the side of the kitchen.

Finally, after months of brainwashing and begging by me, Dad and Mum eventually gave in and we all caught the bus up to Guide in Blackburn, where there was a dog rescue centre. The day before a litter of puppies had been born and I was in my element as I chose a small cross between a Border Collie and a Labrador.

He was pitch-black with a white cross at the front of his chest. He hadn't opened his eyes and I still remember the first time I held him, over the moon that I finally had a dog. Luckily for me, as I was holding him he opened his eyes for the first time; everyone was excited that I was the first thing he saw.

We brought him back home a few weeks later, with me carrying him in a small light-blue school bag with his head popping out the top of it. We named him Mac and for years he was to become a central part of our family.

I took Mac everywhere with me, and the daily routine of leaving with Dad in the morning to go to Nan and Grandad's now included Mac. Mum's parents didn't think that a dog was a good idea, but he soon became a favourite of them too, being fed the best offcuts of meat Nan could get from Blackburn Market.

As the years progressed, Dad found a happy balance of contentment at home while continuing to perform in the clubs and pubs, with the occasional singing job in old folks' homes or charity shows. It could be said that he made peace with the fact that this was his 'fame' and that was OK.

Saturday nights would see Mum and Dad go dancing at the Lion's Den in Little Harwood, while on Sunday afternoons we'd all go up to the Ooozebooth Inn at the top of Oak Street in Blackburn. It would be packed with people eating, drinking and singing along to the jukebox – probably just like The Cora was back in Wednesbury.

When I was around 6 or 7, Dad had a gig at the Blakewater Lodge home for the elderly at the bottom of Whalley Range. While he was practising at home he taught me and my friend Ellen a couple of songs – 'Roses of Picardy' and 'Milly Molly Mandy' – which it was decided we would sing in his show.

Ellen wore her best dress, which I remember was blue and looked a bit like something Dolly Parton would wear, while Mum got me a navy-blue suit from Blackburn Market. All of us walked down from Cedar Street, through Bastwell and down Whalley Range to the old folks' home. Both myself and Ellen carried a small suitcase, which at the time seemed ginormous, but in reality were probably the size of a small book. In them we had our 'music' and lyrics – thinking we were about to do the performance of our lives.

The home had even given us our own dressing room; we thought we were the stars. While Dad was onstage singing we were playing around when out of nowhere a man dressed as the Invisible Man came into the room, scaring us on purpose. He had toilet roll around his face, black glasses, a suit and a bowler hat. We were terrified and ran screaming through the home – which at the time seemed a warren of corridors – straight onto the stage where Dad was performing. Everyone was in hysterics laughing.

After performing our songs onstage, our job was then to go around to all the residents topping up their drinks. All the old people were plastered by the end of the night.

In the early 1980s Dad joined a group called The Versatiles, made up of three women, a male piano player and him, who did charity shows around Blackburn and Darwen. At the time, I thought the two old women in the group were Hinge and Bracket, a famous drag act on TV at the time. Dad would often take me along and I would sit in the audience or play backstage at venues ranging from the Darwen Library Theatre to old folks' homes at the edge of town. Either way, I would be fussed over constantly by all the old women who came to see the shows and who would shower me with sweets.

As a child, it felt like showbiz was everywhere and that everyone's dad was onstage like mine – so much so that I ended up thinking that the family of five girls who lived next door to my nan and grandad were The Nolans, my teacher at school (Mrs Scholes) was Princess Diana at the weekend, and – after seeing a photo of her with long black hair – my mum was Wonderwoman before I was born.

In 1984, Nan told Mum about a woman who had sadly passed away up the road from her. She had no children and the house was going cheap for a quick sale. 'There were two houses just doors from one another,' Mum says. 'But when we looked through the back bedroom window and saw the garden we both fell in love with the place.'

The house on Whalley Old Road in Sunnybower, is a small semi-detached house, just up the road from where Nan and Grandad lived. When they moved in there were red-brick walls at the front of all the gardens and lots of trees – all of these gradually disappeared as people bought cars and put in driveways. The back garden was overgrown, with two huge greenhouses right at the back and a shed that me and my friend Jason would hide in. Inside, the house hadn't been decorated in years; it needed a lot doing to it. Behind the garden was a massive field with overgrown allotments and a small stream. Coming from Cedar Street, I thought this was heaven and I'd bring the other kids up from there to come and play.

After buying the house, Mum and Dad would spend every weekend doing it up, moving belongings from Cedar Street up to Whalley Old Road in a wheelbarrow every Saturday morning.

I have many memories of us all walking up Laburnum Road, Dad wheeling the barrow full of pots or whatever they decided to move that day, Mum carrying plastic bags full of clothes and me and Mac walking behind. The day the big move came, I was able to sit in the back of the removal van. I can remember it to this day. It was bright white, stuffed full of all our furniture, and I was sat on top of some drawers. I remember the shutters coming down and then being tossed around in the back of the van surrounded by all the furniture from our house – a Health and Safety nightmare.

The summer felt like it went on for ever. We'd spend the weekend in what then seemed like a mansion, me and my friends playing in this huge overgrown garden, exploring the fields at the back and climbing into Premier where Dad worked and looking at the Page 3 girls that the men had pinned to the walls of the offices.

Because there was no cooker, most nights we ate soup, bizarrely heated over an old fondue set Mum had picked up. Dad continued his theme of being terrible at DIY and so he was kept away from anything important. Grandad did most of the wallpapering, while Dad chopped back the garden and demolished the old sheds. For years they always seemed to be decorating or doing something in the garden. Dad pulled down the old wall at the front of the house to make way for a drive to park the car. I'd help mix the concrete while our dog Mac would be sat on top of whatever bits of wall remained.

In the midst of all this, Dad tried to teach me to sing. A friend of my mum's had a son who was the same age as me and wanted to be a popstar when he grew up, so it was arranged that once a week he'd come round to our house and Dad would give us singing lessons. It was a disaster. Dad would spend ages showing us how to sing and perform the songs, then say, 'Right, you practise this, and I'll be back in a bit.' Then, he would go into the other room to watch football on TV. The other kid wasn't interested in any of the songs Dad gave us to sing. He'd wanted to learn *Wham Rap!*, not the George Formby numbers that Dad was teaching us. Whilst the other kid sat on the sofa sulking, I pranced around like I was in the West End, singing *Leaning On a Lamp Post* or *When I'm Cleaning Windows*. It didn't last long.

I wouldn't say Dad was the most textbook of fathers. There was no 'bonding' by being taken to football matches, no particular father-and-son time. He got on with doing his own thing – which was singing. But when things mattered he was there, and I never felt unloved or uncared for. Despite the arguments between Mum and Dad, there was always a lot of laughter and love in the house. Dad would often have us in stitches with impressions of people he'd met, while Mum would flounce around the house pretending to sing and dance (painfully) like Kate Bush, or whoever she'd seen on *Top of the Pops* that week. It was an idyllic time, and I felt safe and secure. Then came my teenage years, though, and with them, a whole new set of complications.

Puttin' On The Ritz

Dad and I were very different. Looking back, after leaving Cedar Street and moving up to Sunnybower, I made very few new friends and I became quite shy. I secretly wanted to be as confident as my dad, and if I'm honest, I was desperate to be like he was onstage. But it wasn't meant to be, mainly as I lacked his ability not to give a damn about what people thought. On top of this, puberty was beginning to kick in, which made everything feel a hundred times worse. I was conscious that I was different from the other boys in the class, but at the time I didn't know why. Despite being picked for the school football team, I would freeze when we had to play any matches. This wasn't helped by the fact I ruined my kit before I'd even had the chance to play a single match – I was so excited I decided I wanted to iron it myself, with disastrous results. I remember taking out the iron, plugging it in and plunging it onto the front of the shirt, which immediately melted the polyester into huge strands of plastic. 'Daaaaaaad!' I screamed and spent the next hour in tears. Mum sewed up the hole, but it meant that my shirt was lopsided, literally hanging down to my knees on one side, while on the other it was higher than my waist. The team got into the schoolboy finals playing at Ewood Park, but while every other boy in the side was excited about running on the pitch, I was drowning in dread and distracted at the state of my kit, constantly trying to pull it down as I anxiously ran around.

Dad would come and watch me play but never seemed that impressed with my performance – and who could blame him? I remember him standing on the other side of the railings at the back of the field at Roe Lee School, shouting: 'For Christ sake, Simon, PASS IT!'

Given how good he and his brothers had been on the pitch in their childhoods, how much time and energy they'd all given it and how proud Maurice had been of them, it didn't take a genius to work out that he wouldn't be turning cartwheels at my lack of skill. He would try and concentrate on the positives as we walked home ('You're bloody fast, Sime – you just need to learn how to kick it...') but I think we both knew I was a lost cause. Afterwards Dad told my nan and grandad, 'He runs around like a blue-arsed fly. He chases the ball, gets it, then panics', which was a polite description of how I looked on the pitch, but hearing that just reinforced the fact I felt I was letting everyone down.

I knew I was different from the other boys at this time, but I also felt like I wasn't a son my dad could be proud of. This just intensified my feelings of inadequacy, especially as football had the potential to be the one thing we could bond over – it certainly wasn't going to be music as I couldn't sing anything like him and didn't have the confidence to be onstage, despite secretly having the same desire. For some strange reason, I thought that if I told anyone about wanting to sing, I'd be labelled a 'poof' and be laughed at. I know that Dad had looked up to his own dad because of a shared love of football and singing and that he was proud to have been nurtured by him, so it makes me feel sad that I had built this invisible wall around myself, trying to prove to him and everyone else who I thought I should be.

Despite the fact I didn't feel I lived up to his expectations, Dad would always stand my corner. I saw him in action one night at the school parents' evening when I was in Year 6 – I was waiting outside the classroom when he suddenly stormed past me, slamming the door as he left, shouting 'Come on, Sime, we're going!' I had no idea why he was so cross (I knew not to ask questions when he was in a mood like that) and ran behind him as he marched out of the school. Years later, he told me that the teacher had said I wouldn't amount to anything. He then told the teacher, 'Maybe so, but whatever he does, he'll still be better than you.'

After leaving primary school I passed the 11+ exam and won a subsidized place at the local grammar school, Queen Elizabeth's, or QEGS, which was 500 years old and one of the best schools in Lancashire at the time. Dad was proud. Mum's brother, my Uncle George, had gone there too, so when Dad went down to tell my nan and grandad that I'd got in, Nan ended up dancing around the living room. But going there from Roe Lee Park was a massive culture shock – most of the teachers at the time wore gowns and old-fashioned mortarboards on their heads, and they took sport very seriously.

It's fair to say I didn't have the relationship I wanted to with Dad when I was at secondary school. Something had changed and I couldn't put my finger on what it was. He felt distant and often short-tempered about something, and I'd end up taking Mum's side in arguments. Dad also had a big personality – he played for laughs – and, while there were always a lot of laughs, sometimes when we were out, he would focus more on strangers he had just met than the people around him. It was frustrating, but it was easy to see that life at Butlin's would have been perfect for him as he was always 'on'. Back at home though he could easily fly off the handle when things didn't go his way – especially when attempting any job around the house, which invariably ended with him shouting 'COW IT!' at the top of his voice, and hammers and screwdrivers would end up flying across the room.

On Sundays, Dad and I would drive up to Audley in Blackburn where they were demolishing hundreds of Victorian terraced houses. We'd spend hours filling the car with salvaged bricks or old chimneys that Mum would use for flower pots in the back garden. Dad would use a chisel to clean up the bricks and I'd stack them in the back of the Mini Metro as best as I could, with Mac looking on in the background. There were rows and rows of derelict old houses, but one still had windows and its front door intact. 'There'll be some good stuff in here,' Dad said and proceeded to try and break down the back gate with a sledgehammer. Suddenly at the upstairs back window, a face appeared. I screamed at the top of my voice, thinking it was a ghost. Dad wouldn't listen to me and continued banging away. Then it appeared again. 'Dad! Dad! It's a ghost! It's a ghost!' I shouted. Dad ran around the front and knocked on the front door, apologizing profusely to a decrepit old man – the last person living on the street. Meanwhile, I was halfway up the road, terrified of who it might be.

Looking back now it makes me sad that we wasted so much time when his head was clear. He had a great sense of fun and was never short of a story. I think about all the conversations we could have had, the laughter we could have shared, where I could have found out more about him and he could have been the one to tell me. It's a perversity of life that only when things are taken away from you are you able to realize how valuable they are. For someone so attached to his dreams, Dad also turned out to be an exceptional carer. That's something I remember now as Mum and I both care for him.

Dad lost Maurice and Hilda suddenly, but my mum's parents aged slowly in front of our eyes. One lunchtime in 1988, Dad popped round to Nan and Grandad's on his lunch break. By now their relationship had developed into a deeper understanding and affection towards each other. Nan was endeared by his quirky ways; he enjoyed their closeness. As both were avid readers, he would often bring round books that he thought she would like or small gifts. But when he got there that he found that Nan was ill in bed. This was a big shock as she was never ill. The doctor came round and couldn't seem to find anything wrong with Nan, instead diagnosing her with 'exhaustion', which in hindsight was ridiculous, given how tough my Nan was. I was still going to Nan and Grandad's after school for tea, but now in the evenings Nan would sit next to me on the sofa with a big bucket from under the sink. Every now and again she would leave the room and be sick – one time I saw her standing with her head over the kitchen sink throwing up and I felt terrified at seeing my strong nan looking so frail.

Things slowly got worse and Mum and Dad became concerned. Mum looked worried all the time and went to see Nan every day after work. One night a few weeks later she came home after visiting and we immediately knew something was wrong. She sat there in silence as Dad served up the tea and she picked at her food. Eventually he asked her what was wrong and she just burst into tears, saying sadly: 'She's just given me her engagement ring.' It was clear to everyone that Nan obviously knew she didn't have much time left.

On the weekend of Nan and Grandad's fiftieth wedding anniversary, we all went down to the Three Fishes pub in the Ribble Valley. Mum's older cousin Mavis and her husband Jack came over from Stockport to celebrate. Just as we sat down, Nan got up to go to the toilet. After about ten minutes we were all sitting there, wondering where she was. Suddenly, a man came over to our table looking worried.

'Is that old woman with the red hair with you lot?' he asked.

'Yes she is,' said Mum.

'She's sat outside being sick.'

It was the earthquake that was to shake the foundations of my childhood.

Mum and Dad jumped up from the table and the next thing I remember is an ambulance being called and us leaving the restaurant without eating a thing. Nan was taken to Blackburn Royal Infirmary and she stayed there for a few nights while we waited to get test results and find out what was making her so ill.

One night we all went in to see her – me, Mum, Dad and Grandad – and tried to cheer her up as best we could. As we said our goodbyes, the doctor appeared and took Mum and Grandad into a side room while I sat outside with Dad. When the door opened Mum was bawling her eyes out and Grandad just looked blank.

'They say she's got three months,' Grandad said.

We all got into the Mini Metro in silence, Grandad and I in the back and Mum and Dad in the front. We stopped at the top of Tintern Crescent, just opposite Grandad's house, to drop him off.

'Why don't you come to ours tonight, Dad?' Mum said.

'I'll be fine,' he replied, and then put his arm over his face and started sobbing for what seemed like hours. I didn't know what to do as I'd never seen my grandad cry before; watching him cry for Nan set us all off, apart from Dad who consoled Mum.

Nan died in winter that year, a week before my Uncle George, his wife Sylvia and my two cousins, Kate and Rachael, came over from Australia. Even though George was devastated that he hadn't been able to see his mother before she died, his arrival was just what we all needed – we spent time as a family reminiscing about Nan – sharing stories, sitting up late, laughing and crying. Dad was great, as he always was in a crisis – he could take the edge off any stressful situation by being exceptionally caring and kind.

But I felt the gulf between myself and Dad was growing bigger by the week. I showed no interest in sport or singing, at least not out-wardly so we had very little common ground besides the greenhouse effect or politics, which we'd argue about.

While I was buried in books upstairs in my bedroom, trying to be the best in every subject I could, Dad would be singing his heart out in the front room, blowing the ceiling off as he sung what I thought were old-fashioned songs for hours on end, stopping and starting records as he went over the lyrics. I'd shout down to him to turn the volume down or have meltdowns to Mum that it was driving me nuts as he practised 1930s music-hall songs for any shows he had coming up that week. When he finally did emerge from the front room, it would be in a cloud of smoke from the cigarettes he'd constantly have on the go. 'Tonight, Matthew, I'm Eddie Carter,' Mum and I would joke.

We'd sit down to watch *Top of the Pops* together every Thursday, but as soon as it started, we'd have a falling-out when he criticized everything that came on. 'Gerroff!' he'd jeer at the TV while Technotronic mimed to 'Pump Up the Jam'. 'Call that music! It's just a bloody racket!'

The one thing I did know he was proud of was my grades at school. I knew that QEGS was the opportunity for me to excel, a stepping stone to getting a good career, helping Mum and Dad out financially and making them proud. So I worked as hard as I could and at the end of each term I would come home with glowing reports and top of the class, which Dad would tell everyone at the factory about.

I used to wonder if Dad had always found everything so easy. He wasn't afraid to talk to anyone and seemed to have bags of confidence, while I was painfully shy. It was particularly obvious at family parties – massive events where they'd have to hire out school halls because of the numbers. Dad would be chatting to everyone, and without fail he'd end up singing a few numbers along with Uncle Fred. Meanwhile I'd be sat frozen at a table, scared to speak to anyone. The whole family was outgoing and sociable, but Dad just shone.

At the same time, going to QEGS I felt like I was surrounded by boys from wealthy backgrounds. When I first started at the school there were a couple of them who were talking about their dads owning companies, so I made up an entire story about how Dad owned Premier. Little did my classmates know he worked there as a machinist. I was never embarrassed about him or my family, I was just worried about not being part of the group. Meanwhile, on the public bus on the way back home, other schoolkids would call me 'posh' or a 'snob' because I went to QEGS. It was a confusing time – it felt like I didn't fit in anywhere, despite my best efforts.

This awkwardness continued throughout my secondary school

days and wasn't helped by Dad doing more shows locally to bring in some extra money. He started focusing on retirement homes and did a show at one home owned by the mum of one of the boys at school.

'Oi! Is your dad a singer?' he shouted one lunchtime.

'No, he's a stripper. What do you think?' I said, thinking I was being funny.

It was a huge mistake. He was part of the smoking group and had a mouth on him. Lee laughed then walked away and I knew straight away that what I said would go right round the school. Indeed, by lunchtime the next day the news had spread that my dad was a stripper. Disaster!

I guess as a young teenager all you want to do is fit in with the norm, which, ironically, is something Dad had never sought or thought about. Not caring what people think is a trait that I wish I'd inherited; it certainly would have made my school days easier to handle. I was so embarrassed about Dad being a singer and, looking back now, I have no idea why as it was more exciting than working in an office all day. If I could go back now, I would shout it from the rooftops. I must have been 12 or 13 at the time and during one music lesson, Mr MacKenzie, the music teacher, went around the room, asking each of the boys what musical instrument our parents played. There were oboes, flutes, pianos and saxophones. As it was getting closer to my turn I just wanted the ground to open up.

'Nothing, sir,' I said and the class all sniggered. 'They don't play anything.'

The teacher calmed everyone down and the lesson continued.

Afterwards, I was walking alone through what was called the ginnel – a small path through the school – to my next lesson when the music teacher came bounding up behind me.

'McDermott, there's nothing wrong with your parents not playing any instrument. What else do they do? Do they play sport?'

'Well, my dad sings…' I said.

'What! Why didn't you say anything?'

'Because it's not a musical instrument,' I said.

'McDermott, that's one of the best musical instruments anyone can play. You should be proud.' And he bounded off with his cape flapping.

I suppose what I didn't see was how much courage it must have taken for Dad to keep performing, especially as it required him to change with the times and find new ways to keep getting up in front of people. I have so many memories of him lugging all his backing equipment into the back of the red Mini Metro to drive halfway across Lancashire to do a gig. When I think of it now, I just wonder how much courage it must have taken to do that – to suddenly turn up at a place, on your own, set up your own equipment, do an act, including bantering with the audience, sing and then head home. Each time he did it, he would never know what audience was waiting for him.

But things were changing and by the early Nineties, a new reces-sion had hit and money became tight in the venues that Dad would sing in – hardly any of them wanted to pay for musicians any more. Rather than giving up, Dad decided to get some backing tracks made so he could sing along to them. It's not how he wanted to perform but taking his own backing meant he could get more gigs.

Things continued to get tough when Premier closed down and he was made redundant. He'd been there for seventeen years. 'The best job I ever had,' he says to this day. Part of me thinks that this was because it was right outside the back of our house, meaning he could wake up at 7.15 and be there by 7.30. After a few weeks of not working he soon got a job at a firm on Philips Industrial Estate, where he made wooden picture frames. It was an easy job for Dad – I remember him coming back every day with loads of offcuts that he would either use to build something in the shed or burn them on the wood fire.

GCSEs came and went. I got As in every subject, which boosted my confidence during my final year of school. Strangely, just as Dad loved a crowd, I started to enjoy speaking in front of the whole class, which was a massive shift for me. I was spurred on by some fantastic teachers who brought me out of my shell. But A levels were a different matter. I was a good all-rounder but back then we had very little career advice. I confidently told the vice master (yes – that was his title) that I wanted to study all three sciences as well as Maths and English Literature. He was horrible. He stood up from his desk, slammed his hands on the table and bellowed right in my face 'YOU'RE A VERY CONFUSED BOY' and told me to get out. That was the extent of my careers advice. A week or so later I was sitting on a bus next to a boy from the year above. 'What are you doing for A levels?' I asked. 'German, English and Economics,' he said. My friends were doing German, I loved English and with Economics I thought I'd be sorted financially. So that's what I chose. How wrong was I!

It was a disaster. I'd never done Economics before and the teacher had a dislike for me, often singling me out as 'the posh boy', loudly announcing 'Here's the Green Welly Brigade' whenever I'd answer a question, which was ironic really, considering my background. I'd been a swot all through school, trying to do my best, never ever getting less than a B. But at the end of the first term in Year 11, despite gaining As in my other subjects, I obtained an E for Attainment and U for Effort in Economics. I knew full well my dad would go ballistic when I went home.

And he did. He screwed the results into a ball and threw it right back at me. 'What the pissing hell is this?' he said. My confidence took a nose dive – education had been the foundation of my self-esteem. When I felt like I failed in that area, it was as if the ground beneath me had crumbled, leaving me adrift and unsure of myself. It went on for years. Then, in the middle of it all, I started to think that I was probably gay, despite hanging round Blackburn town centre every Friday night, trying to pull girls. I had no idea how Dad would react if he knew the truth, so I ignored the reality and carried on trying to be the son I thought he wanted.

There's Nothin' Like a Dame

When I started at university in Manchester, I rarely went home, and when I did, I'd spend my time going out clubbing at Peps or Manhattan Heights in Blackburn or working down town at a disco-bar called Toffs.

I was more preoccupied with my own life than what Mum and Dad were doing. At university, I was a Britpop kid emulating Jarvis Cocker by wearing jumble-sale clothes and dancing like I was having a fit. It felt like there was a gulf between me and Dad – I don't think he knew what I was studying or where I lived half the time, but it didn't really bother me – I was just moving forward with my own life. It's not that we didn't get on, we were just like ships in the night and hardly talked in depth about anything any more.

At Manchester I met Oliver, Rob, Emma, Ro and Jo, to name but a few, and they all became my good friends. They got on with Dad like a house on fire. 'Your dad's great, Si!' they would always tell me. I couldn't see it at the time. I think perhaps part of the problem was that when he was great with everyone else, it only highlighted the relationship that I felt we didn't have. They all loved that Dad sang and still did the occasional charity gig. One of the biggest ones was for the 50th VE Day Celebrations at King George's Hall in Blackburn in the summer of 1995. He did one of his famous medleys and it brought the house down. At the time, though, I thought it was all naff and outdated and all I could see was others getting his best side. I thought I knew it all, but in reality I knew nothing about life, or him.

Dad continued to do the occasional gig at old folks' homes around Blackburn. In those days his shows were less about him having the limelight and more about providing entertainment to those who needed it. He wouldn't charge much – he never did learn that lesson about making money from his music – but he didn't care as long as he was singing. There was one Easter in particular, at an old people's home in Accrington, where Dad's singing blew the place down. All the residents ended up getting drunk and there was an Easter bonnet parade. One lady who hadn't spoken to anyone for months got up and started singing and dancing. She was having the time of her life when, dancing the conga with a party hat on her head, she suddenly collapsed backwards: she was dead.

Dad was devastated that someone had died at one of his shows and apologized to the woman's family, who were also there. 'Don't worry, mate – she hadn't moved from that chair in months! She died having the time of her life. Thank you,' the son said. Dad was booked to come back for their summer party.

His musical knowledge was vast – he could go way back to the 1920s and 30s and had a massive selection of backing tracks that he made from old records he'd pick up from car boot or jumble sales. I used to hate it. Some of these songs felt so twee and old-fashioned. I didn't see how spectacular it was that my dad could remember the words of so many songs from so many eras. He had an encyclopedic knowledge of music and during his sets would often recount the stories behind the song and the singer, captivating the audience. But, surrounded by a backdrop of Britpop and Hi-NRG dance music, to me Dad was just uncool. I had no idea.

One of the old folks' homes Dad sang at offered him the job of in-house entertainer. He would do a few days a week, chatting to the residents and performing some shows. He loved it, as did the residents.

But over time, he became upset by what he saw as a lack of care and attention – probably because they were under-resourced – so he started making a list of what was going on:

- 'Patient left calling for help – no nurses answering.'
- 'Patient's clothes thrown across room and left there all day.'
- 'Patient left in wet bed clothes all day.'

Dad mentioned this to the manager. A week later they said they didn't need him to work there any more.

Mum had also begun to cut down the number of hours she was working so they could go on much longer summer holidays, taking themselves to a mobile home in France. They loved it. It reminded them of their courting days, driving around with the trailer attached to the back of the car, windows open and singing songs. Dad would talk to anyone and everyone and soon they had a fantastic circle of friends – Gloria and Alan, Derek and Pauline.

It was a great time for Mum and Dad – they didn't have to worry about money or work much and could just laze on the beach during the day or go out dancing at night in one of the many beach bars. Despite Dad not being able to speak French, in typical Dad fashion, he'd often manage by acting everything out. They also got to know Francis – a French guy who played piano and sang in the Octagon bar on the beach. Of course he couldn't speak a word of English but they ended up communicating – though each of them could have been having a completely different conversation for all they knew. One night Francis let Dad sing and it was like he'd stepped back in time to his Butlin's days. After that night he always called Dad, 'Mon ami

Edward', and Mum and Dad would always get fussed over whenever they arrived at the bar.

Dad hadn't lost any of his shine onstage and one summer stands out. There was a French performer onstage, in a big white suit, face covered in dark fake tan, a gold medallion hanging down his chest, singing terribly and ruining the Rat Pack classics. He was weaving his way through the crowd, encouraging people to join in with his song.

'Please don't come near us, please don't come near us,' I prayed to myself. I hated the attention that Dad could attract in these situations and I just knew what was about to happen.

Dad sat there quietly in his chair, taking the occasional sip of wine, and I could see him smiling quietly to himself. The singer came dancing over to our table, singing the Louis Prima classic 'Just a Gigolo' but in French and leaning into our seats. As he popped the microphone in front of Dad's face, there was no doubt that he was trying to show us up, thinking Dad wouldn't know the song. But Dad took the mic and responded by singing the next line in perfect French. The guy's face dropped and he invited Dad to get up onto his feet and finish the song on his own. Dad had upstaged everyone. The audience all stood up and started clapping and cheering and we were then brought a round of drinks on the house. Despite cowering in my chair and dying of embarrassment, I felt quiet pride for my dad, even if I didn't want to show it.

It was a happy time for Mum and Dad. Their arguments had finally ceased to be as dramatic as they'd been when I was growing up. Dad had acquired an old bike from one of his friends on the campsite, and used to cycle down to the shop every morning to buy baguettes. Other days, Mum and Dad would take the boat over to St Tropez and shop at the market, buying vegetables, living the Riviera lifestyle. They were happy days and ones I know my mum looks back on with great affection.

But they weren't to last. Out of the blue, Grandad was diagnosed with lung cancer. It was a blow, as he seemed to have started to rebuild things after Nan's death. Much like Hilda after the death of Maurice, when Nan died, Grandad had isolated himself and shied away from his friends as he sat at home dealing with his grief on his own. But Mum persuaded him to go back to dancing and there he met Gladys. It was fantastic to see him come back to life again and we were glad when they married. Grandad's illness, however, meant that Gladys found it increasingly difficult to look after him, so it was decided that he would come and live at Mum and Dad's.

During this time, Dad was Grandad's main carer. He cooked for him while Mum was working and would take him for drives out in the countryside. They became very close. The irony isn't lost on either Mum or me that Dad was a true star when anyone was ill. He could be incredibly caring and thoughtful and, when patience was required, he would always step up. It's hard to forget the hours he invested in Grandad and how he just got stuck in because he hated seeing anyone in distress.

Towards the end of his illness, Grandad became more and more confused. I'd often sit with him while he'd try to call up people on the TV by using the remote as a telephone. It was an upsetting introduction to an illness we would end up knowing far too much about.

Grandad died in the spring of 2000. On the day of his funeral Dad did a reading on behalf of the family while I read 'If' – a poem by Rudyard Kipling that Grandad always had hanging in the hallway of his house. It felt like the end of an era with the death of my grand-parents and it triggered something in me.

I couldn't keep lying to Mum and Dad about who I was. I felt I was living two separate lives: one down in London with the occasional boyfriend, and another life up in Blackburn with questions about girls and who I was dating. I felt like a fraud and I hated lying to my parents – it's something we had never done as a family. I'd meet people in London, other gay men, who'd tell me how they didn't speak to their families any more and I didn't want that to happen to me – I didn't want them going to their graves not knowing who I was.

As I mentioned earlier, I think I always knew I was different from a young age – probably around 8 or 9. Dad, like most men of the time, wouldn't think anything of calling someone a 'poof', 'shirtlifter' or 'queer'. (The irony being that, having worked in showbiz all his life, he probably came across scores of gay blokes – and without doubt he wouldn't have treated them any differently. It was drummed into me that I had to treat everyone the same, no matter who they were or where they came from.)

I remember being in my early teens and Mum and Dad were angry about something. 'Your dad's upset because Terry at work said that he thought you were gay,' she told me. I don't think I even knew what the word meant at the time but it was ingrained in me that being gay was wrong, and not something to shout about.

For months I thought about telling Mum and Dad, but just didn't know how to do it – I was terrified of the upset I knew it would cause them. At the same time I was stuck in an admin job in London. When I first got to the city I went to a series of auditions for bands, bringing out the Jarvis Cocker-style persona that I'd created during university. I didn't tell anyone, and would traipse around to backstreet studios to audition. I knew I wasn't as good a singer as my dad but I wanted to give it a go. It was a disaster and I cringe about it now. But, like Dad, my life took an unexpected twist when I saw an advert in the paper: 'Can you sing and dance? Do you speak German/English/Spanish?' The auditions were that lunchtime. I was bored out of my mind in the job and knew I had to make a big change. I spoke a bit of German, knew a bit of Spanish, so I left the office and headed over to a hotel in Victoria, where the interview was completely in German. The guy showed a few videos of the shows and what we were expected to do and asked me if I thought I could manage that.

'Yeah, I can give it a try,' I said.

'Great. Training starts in six weeks,' he replied.

Six weeks later I found myself in Mallorca as a 'Starfriend' at a chain of German hotels, teaching sports during the day and taking part in shows at night. It was bargain-bucket Butlin's – hard work, but I loved it. I knew I had to deal with being gay, so with the safety of living abroad and before I lost my nerve, I took myself off to Palma to finally write Mum and Dad a letter and tell them how I felt. I sat in a cafe writing and crying so much the waiter started to top up my coffee cup for free. I was terrified they would disown me. Two hours later, I put the letter in an envelope, added the stamps and dropped it in a post box opposite. 'You've done it now, Simon,' I thought.

And then I waited.

About three weeks had passed and I heard nothing. Eventually I called them. Dad answered, chatting away as if nothing had happened. 'Dad, did you get a letter?' I asked him.

'Oh, that. Yeah, we did. It's your life, Sime. You've got to do what makes you happy. It doesn't bother me.'

I felt a huge relief.

Mum came on the phone and it was a different story. Her first worry was that I would be wearing make-up and women's clothes, something that Dad and I would laugh about on the phone later. 'You know she thinks you're going out in dresses?' he would tell me. 'Oh, my God! Seriously?'

Only a few years later did she make peace with me for being gay. 'I would never have turned you away for being gay. I was just upset because I thought people wouldn't speak to you and you'd be all alone,' she told me. But little did she know far bigger things were about to test her.

By the time Dad was 65, Mum had noticed that his memory wasn't as good as it used to be, although she didn't mention anything to me at the time. She used to make a joke of it by saying things to Dad like: 'Either you're not listening to what I'm saying, you're ignoring me or you're losing your memory.' But no one thought anything of it. I suppose you don't when life is busy – it's harder to notice small changes when you're with someone every day. Around the same time, whenever Dad would go to gigs to set up his speakers, Mum began to notice that he would get more and more annoyed with himself. Dad's short temper wasn't anything new. Mum was used to his 'artistic temperament' – after all, it had been the cause of so many of their fights in their early days together. But this was different, because it was irritability coupled with a lack of confidence in what he was doing.

When Dad stopped gigging altogether it should have signalled that something was seriously amiss. Yet even then we didn't twig. He would get so stressed beforehand it just wasn't worth it. I'd get the occasional phone call from Mum in tears because of his unreasonable behaviour, but by this time I was getting fed up and thought it was more of the same. 'Mum, if it's that bad, just leave,' I would tell her. However, as usual, the next minute they'd be best friends again. We had no idea then that the illness was making everything so much more intense.

Despite my irritation, I decided I wanted to surprise Dad with a trip to London. I planned the weekend: we would go to different music clubs, including Ronnie Scott's, as I knew he would love the live music. It was also another attempt to try and connect with him – I loved him dearly, but we seemingly had nothing in common and I was clutching at straws to think of something we would both enjoy.

So, I bought a train ticket for Dad, telling Mum to pack him a bag and not say anything. On the day of the trip I called Dad and he told me he wasn't coming, that we would have to do it another time. In hindsight, this was almost certainly due to his fear about travelling on public transport alone. A trip to London would have seemed insurmountable when he couldn't even remember a conversation he'd just had.

Before long, it was Dad's seventieth birthday. All my aunties and uncles from the Midlands had come up to celebrate with him, and we had a big family meal in a hotel in the Ribble Valley. After we'd all said our goodbyes, Mum, Dad and I sat in the car, ready to drive home, and Dad suddenly went silent, looking down at the steering wheel.

'You OK, Eddie?' Mum asked him.

Dad quietly started to cry. 'I'm OK. I just think that could be the last time I see them all together,' he said.

'Aw, don't be daft!' said Mum, giving him a hug.

And he turned on the engine and drove home. It was like he knew something was on its way.

Fings Ain't Wot They Used T'Be

By 2011, life seemed on track. I was living in South Africa with my then-partner, Johannes. It was all about the gym and the beach and I was working remotely as a content editor for an ad agency back in the UK. Life was good. Mum and Dad seemed happy back in Blackburn, even if Dad was a little forgetful.

Johannes and I had moved across the globe to be closer to his mum, who had memory problems. When she came to stay with us in our house, I had my first insight into what it was like living with someone who was confused and forgetful. While Johannes was out at work she would ask me five or six times an hour what time it was. It didn't really bother me – she was mild-mannered, calm and happy, and there weren't any outbursts. Often she would just wander up the road looking at the flowers in people's gardens, sometimes sneaking back with a couple of them that she would hide in a drawer. I would keep an eye on things while I was working and got used to her little outings. One afternoon, however, I was doing some work and realized she had been out a lot longer than usual. I walked up the street to check on her but she was nowhere to be seen.

I continued to the main road, looking in all the gardens, but still I couldn't find her. By now I'd gone round to all the neighbours in the street and it was starting to turn to dusk. I was beginning to panic – I'd already driven deep into the woods at the back of the house where the baboons lived and still there was no sign of her. I didn't dare call up Johannes and tell him I'd lost his mum, especially as it was getting dark. A couple of the neighbours organized a small search party while I drove around calling out her name. As I turned onto one of the main streets, I saw a car on the opposite side of the road with a little old lady in the passenger seat, waving happily at me. The woman driving told me she'd found her half a mile away, wandering down a dual carriageway in the middle of nowhere. 'Please don't tell Johannes,' said his mum.

'Don't worry, it'll be our secret,' I said.

He found out a week later when one of the neighbours said to him: 'So they found your mother then!'

I would look at Johannes's mum and think that Dad must be fine – he wasn't as confused as her and was always reading, always switched on, always interested.

Then Mum called me.

'Simon, I think your dad's memory is really going, it's bad,' she said.

'Well, he is getting old, Mum,' I replied, just putting it down to his age. I didn't think it was anything to worry about.

To begin with, I didn't really pay too much attention to what she was saying as I wasn't there to witness it. That was until I flew back for Christmas. At first, everything seemed normal – Dad was his usual self, Mum was rushing around trying to get everything right – we were having our Christmas dinner a week early as I had to fly back, but we were still celebrating. I'd bought and wrapped my gifts, deciding to give Dad a book about Nelson Mandela's speeches. He always loved to read. Like his records, there are literally hundreds of books stashed away in the house. When I was growing up he'd always be reading – primarily history or biographies, despite his love of storytelling he never read fiction.

I was washing up one night and Dad came into the kitchen. 'Who bought that book, Sime?' he said.

'The one about Nelson Mandela? I did, Dad.'

'Oh, it's brilliant.'

Two minutes later he shouted to me from the lounge. 'Who bought this book, Sime?'

I stopped what I was doing and thought he was taking the mick. 'Dad, I bought that book. It's your Christmas present.'

'Oh, brilliant! It's great.'

I carried on washing up and then again, two minutes later, he came back in. 'Simon, who bought this book?'

By this time I thought he was definitely winding me up – which he so often did. 'Dad, are you having a laugh? I bought it for you. For Christmas.' Over the next hour he must have asked me about ten times who bought the book. It drove me daft. That's when I knew something had seriously changed.

This time I booked an appointment with the doctor. Those few days at home had showed me that Mum was right to be concerned: Dad's behaviour just wasn't normal. I went back to South Africa feeling anxious. At the doctor's, Dad was diagnosed with having high blood pressure and put on a course of statins as well as being told to change his diet. He took the tablets religiously, started eating better and made sure each morning he took himself off for a 'power walk' down to the shops in Little Harwood to pick up the paper.

In January 2012, Dad's brother, my Uncle Ernie, died. It was a huge shock, the first one of his siblings to die, and it must have knocked him sideways. He seemed to lose his sense of purpose and started spending hours in the shed at the back of the garden and he rarely played any of his music any more.

We thought that perhaps he was happy spending time by himself, pottering about in the shed, breaking apart old machines and taking the metal to the scrap-metal yard for cash. It wasn't a huge amount of money but it was something. But his behaviour started to become more than unreasonable and Mum would often phone up in tears about things he was doing and saying. Things dragged on and by early 2012, despite having regular check-ups with the GP, nothing had been mentioned about Dad's memory.

When I moved back to the UK from South Africa the first thing I did was to go back home to see Mum and Dad. I had been warned by Mum that things were a mess. When I arrived, I was shocked to find that Dad had nailed down all the windows in the house and outside he'd used his microphone cables to tie up some plants. On top of that, the back garden was full of things that he had collected but was refusing to throw away or take to the scrapyard. It was piled up everywhere – you couldn't move for junk. There were old washing machines, metal tables, office chairs that he'd picked up from skips, old irons, clothes maidens – anything that had a tiny bit of metal on he kept – but nobody was allowed to go near it. If I tried to move or touch anything, he would fly off into a huge rage.

'Dad, why don't we take some of this to the skip and get rid of it?'

'Don't you touch that! I'm taking that to scrap.'

'But, Dad, half of this is plastic – you'll never get the metal out of it.'

'GERROFFFFF!' And he would snatch what I was holding out of my hand. 'Touch this again and I'll break your legs,' he'd say.

This situation went on for a few months, but the threats got worse and worse so we just left the junk where it was. Dad was still driving at the time and would come back with any bit of scrap that he had picked up. It had become an obsession. Eventually the back garden was so full up with junk, and Mum was so fed up with it, that we had to take the situation into our own hands. I knew it would lead to World War Three on the day, but it just had to be done. There was no space anywhere in the garden – it looked like a rubbish dump.

I booked some time off work and organized a skip so we could just throw the whole lot in. As expected, when the skip arrived, he went berserk. Every time I threw something in he would snatch it from me and put it back. I just had to ignore him and carry on as he called me every name under the sun – it was an utter nightmare and I really thought he was going to punch me.

'Dad, I'm doing this so you can have more space. This is all junk – anything metal that you want to take to the yard I'll leave, but anything else we need to get rid of.'

He stormed off. Then about thirty minutes later he came back. 'Do you need a hand, Sime?' he asked. And I passed him some old bits of plastic chairs. The skip was overflowing – but finally all the junk had gone – and so had my furiously angry dad; instead there was a nice old man wanting to help.

Around the same time, I came back one weekend to drive Mum and Dad to Ormskirk, where Mum's old boss, Mr Connor, was celebrating his eightieth birthday. Wherever I was in the room, Dad would keep waving me over, insisting that I talk to different people. Eventually I just ignored him as it was such odd behaviour and I felt embarrassed. I couldn't speak to anyone without the next minute hearing, 'Sime, Sime! Come over here!' It was constant.

The moment came when we all piled into a room to sing 'Happy Birthday'. I was standing next to Dad, Mr Connor was giving a speech and Dad suddenly started complaining that he couldn't breathe. He then turned around to the curtain, grabbed it, held it to his mouth and started breathing through it. It was more than odd behaviour. He then left the room looking white as a sheet and went to sit in the car. At the time, I thought he was hot because there were too many people there, but looking back it was most definitely a panic attack – probably brought on by the fact that he couldn't understand who the people at the party were. My poor dad. Gone was the man who loved a crowd and a social occasion, now he didn't even know who was in the room or why he was there. Things definitely weren't right, but every time he went to the doctor for a check-up, he would come back saying there was nothing wrong with him.

As Dad was deteriorating, Mum decided it would be a good idea to book their usual trip to the south of France to stay in the caravan for a month between May and June. She hoped that a change of scene and some relaxation would bring Dad back to normal. But as soon as they arrived in Port Grimaud, Dad began to have problems with his eyes, which he would rub constantly until they were red raw. On the first day, their friends Derek and Pauline turned up at Mum and Dad's caravan to take them to the supermarket, but Dad refused to go, which was unlike him. He easily became incredibly frustrated. At one point, he was cooking and he ended up throwing a frying pan across the room, narrowly missing Mum. 'Twat it!' he'd shout and everything would be all over the floor.

Mum kept calling me back in London, telling me how Dad was refusing to leave the caravan. To me it sounded like he had some kind of depression – his behaviour just wasn't like him. Of course he could have his moments, but these episodes seemed to be on a different level. In the past, whatever his mood, he always wanted to go out and be around people.

One evening Mum popped round to see an old couple she knew on the campsite for a cup of tea and she ended up bursting into tears about Dad's behaviour. The old guy walked Mum back to their caravan, but after he'd gone, Dad began accusing her of having an affair with him. His aggression was off the scale, so much so that Mum ended up sleeping in the lounge of the caravan so that if he attacked her, she could escape easily. She called me up that night and it was the first time I heard real terror in her voice – she was frightened of her own husband and said it was like living with a stranger. This was not the holiday they usually had and she swore she would never go with him to Port Grimaud again.

On their return to England, Mum continued to try and get Dad to go to the doctor to get his memory checked. Each time she would book an appointment, Dad would come back and just say: 'Nothing wrong with me.' He was a great actor and it was only later that we found out he would go to the surgery and recite long poems he had written and knew by heart. He would stand in the waiting room in front of the patients and receptionists and perform them aloud – one poem was even called 'Hypochondriacs'! He would go to his appointment and perform as if he was stepping on to the stage, mic in hand, and he'd often have the surgery in stitches. Anyone looking in from outside would think there was nothing wrong with him, while back at home it was a completely different story. I don't know what I thought was wrong, but I didn't make the connection with Alzheimer's.

That summer I met John, a medical student from Birmingham.

'You need to get him checked out, Si – this behaviour isn't normal,' he'd tell me.

'But he goes to the doctor, and they keep saying there's nothing wrong with him.'

'You need to get a second opinion. I'm worried about your mum. How is she coping in all this?'

In September, I booked a train ticket to go up and see Mum and Dad. I was forewarned by Mum that the roof in the back room was leaking and that they needed to get it fixed. It had been like this for weeks apparently, but Dad wouldn't let anyone come round and sort it because he said he would do it himself.

When I arrived home and saw the damage I was shocked – the roof had practically collapsed. They had buckets on the floor to collect any water if it rained, but Dad went crazy when I said that we needed to fix it there and then. It had begun to pour down outside and water was coming in through the roof, so I drove to B&Q and bought some tarpaulin, as well as some wood with which to fix it down. Dad was screaming and calling me every name under the sun while I crawled onto the roof, trying to secure the plastic sheeting in the pouring rain. One of our neighbours came round to help and when I took him inside to show him how far inwards the roof had collapsed, he was shocked: 'I'd seen that water had been collecting on it, but I didn't think it was this bad.'

Mum immediately started crying and Dad continued to fume. I was soaked to the skin, covered in grime and ashamed that I'd been away and let all this happen. We booked a builder to come and fix the roof, but as it was turning into autumn, it was impossible for him to do the work because it was constantly raining, so we made do with the plastic sheeting for more months than I want to remember.

One other thing I noticed on this trip home was that Dad didn't sing in the house any more. Years ago, he would constantly be singing – whatever the time of day he always had a song. He'd set up his equipment in the front room and spend hours belting out classics and going through records that he'd bought from charity shops or car boots, but all that had stopped. Not only that, they didn't go to the clubs any more because Dad didn't want to go out. Even music couldn't make him happy and all he wanted to do was sit in his shed or do newspaper quizzes. By August, when I asked him what he wanted for his birthday, he said a collection of brain-training books. In hindsight, he was obviously trying desperately to keep everything together.

Smile

We knew nothing about Alzheimer's disease. We just thought it meant people forgetting things and in no way did we think that Dad's behaviour at home was connected. It was a lonely time for us. As everything was falling apart, we were still trying to get him a proper diagnosis about what was causing all the strange behaviour. Meanwhile, things were getting worse and his rages were impossible to be around. They would come out of nowhere and were full of frustrated emotion. He lost the ability to filter anything and so it came out in a torrent directed squarely at those who loved him and wanted to help him the most.

Mum's mental health was at breaking point. I'd receive awful phone calls and she'd be in floods of tears – often while I was at work. One time she admitted that, out of nowhere, he came into the kitchen in a rage, dragged her out by the hair and threw her on the floor in the lounge. He was unrecognizable as the man who had swept her off her feet by dedicating songs to her, who had been so vibrant and full of life and kindness. Records would be strewn across the house, clothes would be thrown anywhere, but if you moved them at all, it would lead to one hell of an argument because someone had touched his stuff. Mum would be crying constantly. This was not like the old days when they would row on an equal level – there suddenly weren't any rules and she couldn't just go home to her mum to be scooped up.

'I hate him. I just want him to go,' she would sob.

I'd often find her in the kitchen, crying to herself. Then Dad would come in.

'What's the matter with her? Tell her to piss off,' he would rage.

It was an awful time. He was like a monster, and if truth be told, I also wished he wasn't there – he was making everyone's life a misery.

It got so bad that I thought Dad was developing schizophrenia or psychosis because of the extent of the vitriol and abuse. He'd be fine one minute and the next all hell would break loose.

I was so concerned about Mum's safety that I called up the doctor to try and get an appointment for her to talk about what was going on at home with Dad. There wasn't one available, I was told. But I'd had it and I told them I would be coming down anyway and wouldn't be leaving the surgery until someone spoke to us, even if it took all day. I was sick of all the aggression and weird behaviour – something seriously wasn't right and it had become terrifying. Any fun times with Dad had gone and he was clearly very ill.

Luckily, the regular doctor Dad saw wasn't there, so we had an appointment with a locum who was covering. I went in with Mum to make sure she talked honestly about what was going on. The doctor could see something was wrong as soon as we both entered.

'It's about my dad,' I said.

'His behaviour at home is so aggressive and we don't know what to do any more.'

'Can you describe what he does?' she asked.

'He's fine most of the time. He just gets angry,' Mum said.

'Mum, you need to tell everything that's happened. No one can help you if you don't say what's going on.'

'Has he hit you?' asked the doctor.

Mum just burst into tears and was inconsolable. It was horrible to watch.

'Mum, you need to say what's been going on. Everyone's here to help.'

'We've tried to get his memory tested but each time he comes back they say there's nothing wrong with him,' she said, sobbing.

Her eyeliner was now smudged all over her face. She was in a complete state and I couldn't believe it had come to this.

'I'm really worried for my mum's safety,' I added.

'Listen, I'll get him in again and see what we can do.'

When we left the doctor's, Mum sat in the passenger seat of the car crying.

'Mum, you've done the right thing. You can't go on like this. It's not fair on you. Something isn't right.'

'I just feel like I've gone behind his back,' she said through her tears.

'You haven't – you've done this to help him. But you need to look after yourself.'

I was fighting back the tears myself.

We drove home and pretended to Dad that we'd been shopping. Along with Mum, I felt so guilty – like I'd betrayed him and that I'd let him down as a son. But I also knew we needed help. A week or so later, Mum had managed to get a double appointment with Dad at the doctor's on the pretext that they needed to check his blood pressure. It was only at the end of the appointment that they brought up the topic of memory. Dad was – as expected – defensive, but the doctor carried out the necessary tests, and then said that he would book him in for an appointment at the memory clinic.

We heard nothing for months. We called up the doctor time and time again but they said there was a waiting list and that we shouldn't worry. That was in the October – Dad's behaviour at home continued to become increasingly aggressive and difficult for both of us. It was impossible to know if he had any awareness of how he was behaving. At least in the old days he knew when he was being a nightmare,

SIMON McDERMOTT

but this short and violent fuse was on a whole other level and not something he could seem to control or predict.

Luckily, Mum had her friends around her and Edna, her maid of honour, had heard about a meeting in the town hall to talk about dementia and suggested Mum go along with her. 'The whole meeting was about how they were building new homes for dementia patients,' Mum says. 'I put my hand up and said it was all very well, building new homes for patients, but they needed to get the doctors sorted.' At the end of the meeting the chairman came up and spoke to Mum, asking her the name of her doctor. He said he would try and move things forward for us. Having Edna there was a huge support but it felt light years away from the carefree days of Mum and Dad's courtship and their wedding day. When Edna had watched her best friend marry the man she loved, no one could have predicted it would end up like this.

Around the same time, I was talking to my boss at work about the nightmare that was going on at home. His own mother had also suffered from dementia and he was shocked at our situation – he said the specialist had seen his mum one week after their first doctor's appointment. I knew the time had come to take matters into my own hands, so I found the number for the Blackburn Memory Clinic and called them up directly, eventually getting through to someone who could help.

'When did you say your dad's appointment was with the doctor?'

'October – I mean I know there's queues and waiting lists, but it's now March and we still haven't heard anything.'

There was a silence.

'This is really bad. You should have heard something by now – let me take a look.'

I gave Dad's details and waited while she checked.

'Nope. I'm sorry, there's nothing on the system.'

I repeated the information again, giving one of Dad's many stage names.

'Maybe try Ted McDermott, or Thomas McDermott, or Eddie McDermott.'

'No – I'm sorry, you'll need to go back to your doctor.'

I was furious. We'd waited nearly six months for nothing.

I called the doctor straight away to complain and Dad was fast-tracked to the memory clinic, but of course he refused to go at first. Finally, in June 2013, it was confirmed Dad had dementia. It had taken us eighteen months to get this diagnosis and for him to start receiving medicine. To be honest, all I felt was a huge sense of relief – at least we knew what it was now. Once he started taking the medication, it did initially help to relieve some of his aggression and things became manageable for a while – that is until he started refusing to take it.

Pride and a stubborn nature had seen my dad through the knocks of performing, but those traits do not mix well with dementia. Dad insisted that he controlled his tablet intake, but we knew full well he wasn't taking them. Tablets were found all around the house. Just asking him if he'd taken his tablets would lead to a full-on aggressive rage.

That Christmas Day, he came down in the morning with a face like thunder. His deterioration in just a year was painfully obvious. The previous year he had just been repeating questions; this year he complained about everything. Even the gifts we gave him were dismissed, with him tutting and throwing them to one side. Mum was in tears and I hated him for it. When we told him it was Christmas Day he would simply reply: 'I don't care what pissing day it is.' Things were thrown at us, doors would be slammed, Mum would get pushed around. I wanted to punch him, but I thought if I did he would literally try to kill me.

That December I had just bought a flat in London and was

completely broke. On top of that my relationship with John wasn't going well – we'd always bicker (a pattern that was without doubt handed down to me from my parents), even though we'd just got back together again. I'd go up to Blackburn and have Dad constantly threatening or lashing out and, to top it all off, I'd just started a new job. The icing on the cake was when one of my teeth suddenly cracked in half at work, leading to a £500 dental bill. My work was suffering and I'd only been there a couple of months. One Monday morning my boss took me into a meeting room and gave me a list of tasks she wanted done by the end of the week. I was full of cold and it was the final straw. My eyes started to well up and I felt like I was staring into an abyss. Right then, I didn't give a damn about anything. I'd had it. There was a pause.

'Are you OK?' she said.

'Yeah. It's fine,' I muttered.

'Are you sure? You look like you're about to cry.'

'Yep. Nope. Not really. It just feels like everything's going wrong…' And then I explained to her what was going on. She was great. 'Right, take a breath. This doesn't matter,' she said, pushing the work aside. 'My mum went through the same thing with my grandad. I know exactly what you're dealing with.'

I felt pathetic. Normally I'd be able to cope. But no matter what she said or how much she tried to console me, I felt like I'd been run over. I suppose deep down a part of me also felt I wasn't being the man Dad would have wanted me to be. If he had known what was going on, would he have been proud of me and the way I was dealing with things? I couldn't help but feel the answer would be no.

Back in Blackburn, I was increasingly worried by the fact he was still driving. I had so many discussions with Mum about Dad using the car – it really wasn't safe. Whenever we went out driving it would be unbearably traumatic. He would be swearing at every other driver on the road and it was terrifying to be a passenger – a number of times I got out of the car, refusing to drive with him again. I remember one incident where we'd just had a pub lunch one Sunday and Dad suddenly drove on the wrong side of the road. Both Mum and I were screaming at him to get back on the right side, but he wasn't having any of it, screaming back at us: 'I've driven for years. Don't tell me what to do.' In the end, we had to call a mechanic and ask him to tell Dad that the car wasn't fit to drive. We knew he wouldn't accept it from us and it was the only way we could think of to stop Dad getting in the car until we could make an appointment with the doctor. This was serious. Mum made an urgent appointment with the memory clinic, telling them about the situation, but asking them to say that, because of his eyesight, he needed to give up driving. Luckily it wasn't a problem and Dad went along with it and didn't drive again; instead he walked everywhere – a good thing for everyone. It would make him fit as well as keeping him off the roads and we were all relieved that nothing serious had happened – it could have been a lot, lot worse. But Dad's independence had finally gone and we had resorted to asking people to lie to him. It felt like a real line in the sand and I was terrified at how quickly this illness seemed to be sinking its claws into him and the measures we were already having to take to keep him, and others, safe.

One Saturday I drove him to the newspaper shop because it was pouring down with rain and went in with him.

'Bonjour!' he shouted as soon as he entered.

A shy Asian woman in a headscarf was standing behind the counter and two Muslim men with long beards were waiting to pay.

'Right then, what does Linda want again?' he said to me.

'Paper, milk, and biscuits,' I said.

Dad looked at me and said 'thank you very much' in a fake Pakistani accent.

'Now, where the bloody hell are the papers?' he said, again in the same accent.

I was completely embarrassed. By now the two Muslim guys were glaring at us. I rolled my eyes at them, trying to apologize for the inappropriateness of it all, but understandably they were having none of it.

Meanwhile, the woman behind the counter was grinning, as if she was in on the joke.

I grabbed the shopping for Dad and took him to pay. Thankfully, the two men had left. I really thought they were going to kick off.

'How much is it, Mrs?' Dad asked.

The woman priced everything up. 'Two pound twenty,' she said.

'Bloody hell! I hope you're not ripping me off!' said Dad, laughing. 'Is this enough?' He handed her two £20 notes.

'Don't worry, Dad, I'll get this,' I said, and gave the woman the right change.

Then we left the shop.

'Right, I'm gunna walk to the Co-op.'

'OK, Dad, if you do that then I'll drive round and park by the side.'

As Dad walked off, I ran back into the shop. I wanted to ask her about his behaviour, as well as apologize for him. I was mortified.

'I'm so, so sorry. He was only joking. He just gets confused.'

'Oh, don't be daft!' she said in a broad Blackburn accent. 'I know Eddie – he comes in every day. We have a right laugh together.'

'What's he like when he comes in?'

'Oh, he's very confused. He never remembers what he's come in for half the time, so I just walk him round the shop until we remember – it's usually a paper and some biscuits. He gets very confused. But don't worry, I keep an eye on him,' she said.

I was shocked at hearing this. Poor Dad, I didn't know how confused he would be with people in public – it was clear that doing anything on his own was becoming a struggle.

As I left the shop, she shouted again, 'Don't worry!' I wanted to run back and give her a massive hug – I couldn't believe how understanding she had been, especially about him doing the accent, but I knew not everyone would react in the same way. I drove down to the Co-op with tears in my eyes.

When I went inside the Co-op, I found him wandering around again, trying to work out what to buy. I watched him picking up anything but the things he actually needed, muttering away to himself. When we went to pay, Dad just handed over his entire wallet to the cashier. I felt embarrassed for him – he was like a child and it broke my heart.

It was around this time that Mum bumped into her old friend Eileen at the bus stop in town. Mum and Eileen used to hang around together in the Sixties and I remember from old photos Eileen always used to have a big blonde beehive – and she still did! They had drifted out of touch and hadn't seen each other for years, but fate brought them together that day at a time when we were at our most desperate.

Despite not seeing one another for years, it turned out they only lived down the road from each other, with Eileen living at Larkhill flats. A few days later, she called up Mum and asked if she'd like to go to St Stephen's Club with her one night. They were having an open-mic night and she thought it would be good for her to get out. Inevitably, Dad refused to go, so Mum went alone, but the following week he went along and it then became a regular thing – most importantly, once he was there, Dad was in his element and he was soon persuaded by the old crowd to get up and sing. Suddenly he was back in front of an audience – something that he hadn't done for years.

Mum's meeting with Eileen and their trips to the club gave Dad a new lease of life and reignited his passion for performing. Now he had something to look forward to every week and it was the one night of respite Mum got from the madness. Seeing him up there was like taking a time machine back to his heyday – he was confident, swaying to the music, and didn't miss a beat. No one would have thought there was anything wrong with him. He was word perfect and had the crowd, such as it was, in the palm of his hand. You could have heard a pin drop as he sang 'Here in My Heart'. That's when we realized that singing could be the key to controlling things. The stage was his safe place in a world that felt increasingly terrifying and alien to him. With that in mind Mum and I set up the record player in the back room and brought down some of his old records. It was a massive relief when we saw his reaction – he was like a different man. Suddenly he would spend hours selecting records, putting them on, taking them off again and singing away. His voice still sounded as good as ever. There would be a few occasions when he would fly off the handle, throwing a record across the room, but you could tell that he had started to enjoy singing again. His voice had always brought joy and transported people away to another place; now it seemed it was doing the same for him.

I Whistle a Happy Tune

But let's not sugar-coat things – music could only offer a reprieve rather than a cure. By autumn 2014 things at home were getting worse. Dad's rages were becoming more regular and extravagant. One weekend I went up to visit. Mum had gone to bed early, as she was so exhausted, while Dad and I sat and watched TV. Everything was fine. All of a sudden, Dad jumped up from his chair and ran upstairs. I've never seen him run so fast in his life. The next thing I heard all this screaming from upstairs.

'No, Eddie, stop it! Eddie!'

'I'll break every bone in your body!'

I ran upstairs into Mum and Dad's bedroom. Mum was sitting bolt upright, with her hair everywhere, looking completely startled. The bedcovers had been ripped from the bed and Dad was stood there threatening us both. He looked possessed.

'What's happened?' I asked.

'Make sure she keeps out of my sight. I'll throw her through the window if she comes anywhere near me,' he said. He pushed past me and stomped downstairs.

'Did you say anything to him? Did he hit you?' I asked Mum.

'He just came in and grabbed my hair and started shaking my head…' Mum said.

She was in shock. That rage had no logic and it went on for hours.

It was terrifying. Eventually he agreed to go to bed while Mum stayed in the lounge. I hardly slept that night. In the morning, he had no memory of what had gone on the night before, so we just carried on like nothing had happened.

Even though Dad was no expert at DIY, he'd always have a go at building or fixing things, or pottering about in the garden, keeping things tidy. But that all stopped as the illness got worse and things really started to fall apart. I'd gone up to Blackburn another weekend to do some jobs in the garden to keep on top of things. Outside the front door and around the side of the house the paving stones had become mouldy and slippy – I was worried Mum and Dad would fall on them and the last thing we needed now was a broken leg. I went down to B&Q and bought some mould cleaner as well as a new brush to make it all safe. I'd spent about two hours cleaning and brushing outside the house, all the time with Dad standing there, glaring. I knew he wasn't happy about something but I didn't dare say anything as I sensed he would go for me. I was just finishing off when he came storming out of the house, grabbing the brush from me and pushing my chest.

'Piss off! Get out. It's MY GARDEN!'

'Dad…'

'Piss off out of my garden or I'll break every bone in your body,' he added. By now his face was almost touching mine and his eyes made him look possessed.

This wasn't a threat. If I didn't move there and then he'd kill me.

'Fine. Do it yourself,' I snapped and slammed the door behind me. I went into the front room, where Mum was having some tea.

'What's happened?' she said.

'I don't know what I've done. I was just cleaning up to make sure you don't slip…'

All of a sudden the door burst open and Dad came storming into the front room.

'What are you doing here? Get out! Go on, get out! Piss off!'

'Dad, I've spent the whole weekend doing the garden. Why are you having a go at me?'

'You know why I'm having a go…'

I stood up.

'No, Dad – I don't. You tell me why you're having a go at me.'

By this time we were eyeball to eyeball. I was PISSED OFF. He'd been moaning and threatening me all weekend and this was the final straw.

He laughed in my face.

'Piss off, you're nothing! And you know why you're nothing…'

I knew exactly what he was going to say and it terrified me.

'Go on, Dad. You tell me why I'm nothing,' I shouted in his face.

He jabbed my chest with his finger.

'For years I've been ashamed of you,' he said.

My stomach sank.

'Well, go on, then. You tell me why you're so ashamed,' I shouted.

I'd never been so cocky towards him in my life and I knew, any minute, if this continued he'd punch me.

'You're nothing to me because of what you are. I can't tell anyone I know about you. I'm ashamed of you and so is everyone else. So is your mother but she won't say it 'cos she's too soft.'

'Oh, so that's it then, Dad. Because I'm gay.'

Despite being so cocky with him, it was as if my insides had shattered. It felt like my stomach had fallen through the floor. This wasn't like my dad, he normally hated confrontation for the sake of it; if anything, he was a peacemaker and the one always trying to diffuse everything, but this illness made him furious all the time.

'Yeah, because you're gay. And because me and your mum won't have any grandchildren.'

'Fuck off, Dad!'

I'd never sworn at him before in my life.

There was a scuffle between us and Mum pulled us apart.

I went upstairs swearing and slamming all the doors in the house. Dad went out the back to his shed. I was doing everything to make sure things were OK and all I received were constant threats and abuse from him.

Mum came upstairs. 'Simon, are you OK?'

'Yeah, I'm fine, Mum,' I said, pretending it didn't bother me. I knew if I started to cry in front of her, I wouldn't be able to stop. 'I'm just going to go out for a minute. I need to get some air. Don't worry, I'm OK.'

I got in the car, reversed out the drive and drove to the traffic lights. And then it started. Full-on tears. I was utterly devastated. I was sobbing and crying so much that I could hardly see where I was going. I pulled off at the first turning, which was Whitebirk Industrial Estate.

I couldn't understand what was going on. When I first came out to Mum and Dad, the main thing I was worried about was them being ashamed of me and ultimately letting them down. I had kept it hidden for years because, like most gay men at the time, I didn't want to let down the people I loved. When I had told them, Dad was the one who stood up for me the most. He was the one who calmed everything down, always telling me I had to live my life the way I wanted. 'Bugger everyone else, Sime!' he would say. 'You know what's right for you, as long as you don't hurt anyone.'

But that moment, when he said what he did, I felt like everything he'd ever told me was a lie. It broke me. My worst fear had been realized and I felt like I'd failed at the one thing that I didn't want to fail at – to make my parents proud. I cried like I'd never cried before.

After I calmed down, I drove back to the house, dreading what I was going to walk into. I was terrified Dad would fly off the handle again. I felt like I'd been hit by a bus but I was determined not to stand down or let anyone know that what he had said had affected me so deeply.

I opened the front door and went into the back room.

'Sime? Is that you?'

'Yeah, Dad.'

He was surprisingly happy and cheerful. What the hell was going on?

'I've just made some tea. Do you want one?'

Then he popped his head out the door, smiling, without a care in the world.

'I got some doughnuts from Morrisons so have one if you want. Have you been down town? Was it busy?'

It was like the trauma of the hour before hadn't happened. I couldn't understand it. Dad continued chatting away to me as if he hadn't seen me in ages, and I just sat there like I'd been run over. Nothing else was said and we all continued to live this dysfunctional life.

***

Mum turned 70 at the end of November, so I decided to throw a surprise party for her with the rest of the family. The theme was Dynasty vs France – two things Mum liked – the glamour of the Carrington family and holidaying in France. I didn't tell Dad as I knew he wouldn't be able to keep a secret.

By now he was regularly refusing to go out with Mum, sometimes even when the taxi was waiting outside. She was going through such an awful time at this point, I just wanted her to have one night that was all about her.

I realized that I'd need a Plan B in case Dad refused to leave the house that night, so I enlisted the help of Uncle Colin. Sure enough, an hour before we were about to leave, Dad announced that he wasn't going out. The only thing that persuaded him was the fact that I told him I'd organized some food in a restaurant and he would have a nice meal. He had no idea it was Mum's birthday, which was probably a blessing. Luckily the night was great and Mum loved every minute of it (despite not remembering much after being given too many Jägerbombs by one of my cousins). Everyone turned up in French costumes – wearing strings of onions and garlic and berets. Dad got onstage and sang his songs. For a moment it felt like everything was normal and, at the end of the evening, we filled the taxi with Mum's presents, happy everything had gone so well.

But the next day (on Mum's actual birthday) as she was opening her presents, Dad started saying terrible things to her. We both tried to ignore it. 'Why are they giving her all these cards? I'm the star! She's a nobody.' He was awful. She was sitting around with hundreds of cards and presents – I've never seen so many gifts for one person – but Dad was tutting away and making horrible comments. I knew he was ill, but the nature of this illness is that it plays tricks on you because the person in front of you looks the same way they always have. You forget that the person is ill and you don't understand why they can't control their behaviour. It seemed the ultimate cruelty that Dad could still stand up on a stage and be Teddy Mac, the name that he used down in the Midlands, like he had the night before. He still knew how to do that, but he didn't know how to be decent to those he was supposed to love. It was hard not to think that, yet again, he could turn it on for strangers but not for us. It felt like everyone else had the brilliant Ted stage show, while we had to mop up backstage.

After the disastrous few years we'd had at home, it was decided that Christmas 2014 would be spent at my flat in London. Mum and Dad came down on Christmas Eve and I'd planned a surprise trip to The Shard. We walked down the South Bank and stopped off at a pub on the way for a glass of wine, but Dad was complaining about everything. I prayed that his mood would change as I really didn't want another Christmas to be ruined. A group of workmen were having an after-work drink and Dad sidled up to them, chatting away like he'd known them for years. They were all looking at each other as if he was mad. Dad thought they were kids, and he was talking to them as such. I tried to get him away, as I could sense they would take the mick out of him, but he was having none of it.

'Come on, Dad, come and sit with us.'

'No way! I'm talking to the real stars,' he snapped.

'Simon, just leave him, he won't come back,' Mum said.

So eventually I just sat with Mum with one eye on Dad, watching how the guys were behaving around him. A couple of the younger lads tried to take the mick out of him, but then thankfully the older bloke with them told them to leave it. He looked over and mouthed to me, 'It's OK.' I was so thankful for those simple words. He understood totally what was going on and went along with it, taking my dad to the side away from the rest and having a simple conversation with him.

'Right, I think we need to go and rescue them,' I told Mum.

We put on our coats and wandered over. 'Right, Eddie, we're going now,' said Mum.

'Right, mate. It looks like you'd better go before they all leave you,' said the guy. Dad put on his coat and made his way over to Mum.

'Thanks for that. He gets a bit confused sometimes.'

'Don't worry, mate. I know what you're going through. My father-in-law's the same. I know how it is...'

I shook his hand and walked out. I felt completely humbled – these simple moments of kindness from complete strangers meant so much. Looking back now, Mum and I had felt so incredibly alone in all this, but these occasional simple gestures had been a lifeline to help lift us, momentarily, out of the madness.

We made our way up to London Bridge and to the entrance for The

Shard. After we handed over our tickets we had to pass through an airport-style security gate, so it was the usual procedure – everything had to come out of our pockets, our coats had to be scanned and our belts taken off. Of course, at the time I didn't realize how confusing this would be for Dad. It was a drama to say the least. It took me a good five minutes to explain to him that we had to take our coats off as well as empty out our pockets. The staff looked at us like we had arrived from Mars, smirking at each other. With no idea about Dad's condition, they just thought we were idiots. 'Sorry about my dad – he's ill,' I said. I may as well have been talking to robots – they looked down their noses, full of disdain. Finally, we eventually made it through and then into the lifts up to the viewing floor. Again, I had no idea how much it must have terrified Dad, being up so high. It was a beautiful view and the sun was just setting on a clear day, so the whole city was being shown in its glory. But Dad was having none of it. He got hysterical every time Mum and I stepped towards the windows and wouldn't move from where the lifts were and was literally clinging to the walls.

'Come on, Dad – have a look at the view.'

'Piss off. I'm going!'

He insisted on going straight back into the lift.

I had been desperate for Mum to experience this without any stress, but the whole situation was a nightmare. Dad was shouting at other people around us: 'I don't need to look out of windows. I'm not a bloody sheep, like these twats!' Again, the tourists and the staff were looking at us as if we were the family from hell. Eventually we had no choice but to call it a day and head back to my flat, but I could see the sadness in Mum's face.

Frustration and disappointment became the main features of her life but the old fighting spirit she'd shown Dad when they were dating made a reappearance – she wanted a holiday and she was going to have one. So, in June 2015, despite my reservations and concerns, she booked for her and Dad to return to France.

'I need a life too, you know!' she would say.

It was agreed that they'd go for two weeks in May and I would fly out for about five days in the middle of it, just in case anything happened.

I called Mum on their second night to see how things were and, even though there had already been a huge scene, she sounded calm. I flew out and was surprised to find them both in great spirits. That was until we went for a drink in one of the bars on the site. It was the 'posh' bar, so all the waiters were dressed up and a bit self-important. It was a nice night, so we decided to sit outside.

The first thing I noticed was that Dad seemed to think there were glass partitions everywhere. He was confused, walking towards what was a gap between two pieces of wood with his arm outstretched like he was about to push open a door. And then it started.

'Get me out this pissing place!' he shouted.

'Eddie, calm down,' said Mum.

By now the whole place was looking over. Dad was thrashing about, trying to get out. He then stumbled over a chair, which made things ten times worse. He kicked it, nearly falling over, then stormed out, pushing through the imaginary plate glass door again, and again nearly falling over. We looked like nutcases.

From then on, the holiday got progressively worse. During the day, Dad would be fine – I'd take him along the beach for a walk in the sea and we would chat away, but I noticed that, for the first time, he didn't really know who I was. Most of the time he still called me 'Sime', but he started to tell me stories about Blackburn – stories such as where he worked and that he was the eldest of fourteen children – which obviously he wouldn't be telling me if he knew I was his son.

Everything seemed to suddenly slide – he refused to take any medication, often accusing me and Mum of trying to poison him. I'd sleep in the single bedroom in the caravan, but I could hear Dad insulting Mum when they went to bed. It was the usual stuff – things like telling her to 'piss off' or 'get out of my sight'; all she got was constant abuse and it was horrible to hear. I'd often find her crying to herself, and a couple of times when I did go to console her, he would then lash out at me too, calling me every name under the sun.

The crunch point came when their old friends, Alan and Gloria, invited us all to a bar further along the beach – their daughter was over from London and they'd heard good things about this new place and the entertainment they put on. We ate in the caravan and set off around 7 p.m. to walk to the bar, but I could already sense that Dad was starting to turn. He was moaning the whole way along the beach until we arrived.

'So, what act is on tonight?' I asked.

'Oh, it's an Elvis impersonator,' Gloria said.

I looked at Mum and we both knew this was going to be a HUGE mistake. Dad hates Elvis impersonators, and with the mood he was in, we just knew this wouldn't end well. He had low tolerance at the best of times for people who didn't deserve the spotlight, but this was going to be carnage.

'Oh God,' I thought.

A backing track started and out came 'Elvis' from the stage.

'*Schönen guten Abend*'

It was an Elvis impersonator – but in German.

Elvis was prancing and japing around and the German crowd were falling off their chairs in hysterics. They were loving it. Meanwhile, over on our table Dad was sitting with a furious face on him, like he was about to explode.

'Amateurs,' he kept muttering. 'Fucking twat!' he'd add. Then eventually, 'Nope, I'm going. This isn't entertainment.' Actually, in hindsight, it probably wasn't. It was a nightmare and we ended up having to leave the show early, making a huge fuss as we pushed through all the tables. Dad was practically kicking the chairs out of the way, while me and Mum scuttled behind, apologising to everyone.

By the time we got back to the caravan, Dad was hurling abuse at us. It was pure hatred. 'I know what you two are up to,' he shouted.

'Dad, come on. Calm down.'

It was about 11 p.m. and he was raging on at us at full volume. Everyone in the other caravans could hear.

Mum started sobbing. 'I can't keep doing this.'

'It's OK – we'll sort it out tomorrow,' I said.

I made up the bed for myself in the lounge area while Mum slept in my bedroom, but I could hear Dad pacing and muttering to himself in his bedroom. I had no idea what he was getting up to but it seemed like he was opening and closing cupboards, looking for something. I was terrified – I'd never seen him like this before.

I could hardly sleep, but just as I was drifting off, the door to his bedroom swung open, slamming against the wall. It was around 3 a.m. and by now I was petrified. Although it was my dad, I was scared for our safety. As I pretended to be asleep, I could hear him shuffling around the lounge, still muttering away.

'Fucking swines! Soon as I catch them I'll break every bone in their body. Fucking tea leaves! They think I don't know what's going on.'

I felt like a kid waking up in the middle of the night, thinking there's a monster in the room, and I tried not to breathe or move for fear of making it worse. I heard him opening cupboards and drawers then slamming them shut, and I became terrified he would get hold of a knife and stab us all. Suddenly the shuffling and muttering stopped and there was complete silence. He was standing right over me.

I was sure he was going to stab or at least punch me yet I was completely frozen, preparing myself for the first blow. You would think that I'd have opened my eyes and tried to reason with him but I just couldn't. This was my dad who I knew loved me and I knew wouldn't do anything to hurt me – but that was the old Ted, the man who had been my dad before this illness. I didn't want to acknowledge what was happening – and if I kept my eyes closed, I could pretend he wasn't there. I no longer felt like a man, more a terrified child.

Then it started.

'You fucking toerag!' he growled. 'I know what you've been doing. Fucking thieving, stealing toerag!'

His face was right next to mine.

'I'll. Break. Every. Fucking. Bone. In. Your. Fucking. Body,' he snarled.

Dad rarely, if ever, said 'fuck', so to hear it said with such vengeance directed at me scared the life out of me. It was as if he had become possessed by the devil. The insults went on for about ten minutes or so and then he slowly shuffled back into his bedroom, closing the door behind him. And everything went silent.

'What the fuck just happened?' I thought. My heart was pounding and I lay there staring at the wall of the caravan right in front of me, still not daring to move. I didn't sleep that night at all. Around eightish I heard Mum wake up, so I went in to have a quick chat, telling her what had happened. She started to cry.

'I wish we'd never come on this holiday,' she sobbed.

I made them the usual tea and toast for breakfast, hoping Dad would wake up in a different mood. When he sat down he was a lot calmer, but he still wasn't his normal self. He refused to use anything that Mum touched, and wouldn't sit next to her at the table. He hardly said a thing. In fact, no one spoke apart from a passing comment about what the weather would be like that day. I thought back to breakfast time on holiday when I was small – all the whistling and singing and fun. Here we were, with things so bad that we daren't even speak. What was happening to us?

This same routine went on for the rest of the holiday. We had days on the beach, a nice lunch and Dad would be in a good mood, but by the evening, things would change.

We all wanted to go home but I had no idea how on earth we would get Dad back to England at this rate. The day before I was supposed to leave, I sat in the hire car and called up Uncle Colin for advice.

'You alright, kid?' he said.

'Yes.'

'How's France?'

'Yeah, it's OK… It's just…' my voice faltered, 'Dad.' I started to cry silently.

'You OK, Sime?'

'Yeah, I'm OK.'

'You don't sound OK.'

There was a pause. I desperately wanted to tell him what was going on, but again I felt I'd be betraying Dad and I knew if I spoke I would completely break down.

'Are you there, Simon?'

'It's just Dad. He's getting aggressive again and I don't know what to do…' And then I lost it, crying into the phone.

This wasn't what I wanted to do. I just wanted some advice, I didn't want them to think that I couldn't handle this.

It all came out. Everything that had happened that holiday, I told him.

'I just can't calm him down…

'Sime, whatever you think you need to do, we'll support you all the way. If you need to get him taken away, we'll support you. Don't worry,' he said.

Just the thought of Dad being taken away in a van to a psychiatric hospital set me off crying. I sat in the Port Grimaud Caravan Park with the tears streaming down my face. The fact that I didn't know what to do didn't worry me: it was the fact that no one else seemed to know either.

That night was the same routine and by the next morning I was utterly exhausted. Dad was exactly the same as he'd been at breakfast for the past few days. That morning I cooked some eggs for us, but he again refused to eat them and finally I just let go.

'Dad, what's the matter with you? It's my last day today and you're still acting like this.'

'What do you mean, it's your last day?'

'I'm going back to London tonight. I have to leave at lunchtime to drive to the airport.'

'What? You're going back? Why?'

'Because I have to go and work.'

'Oh, in that case we'd better have a good day then.'

It was like he had suddenly come back in the room and the darkness lifted. I don't know whether it was because he realized I was Simon, but whatever was going through his mind seemed to settle him. Maybe it was because I was leaving! Whatever it was, I felt relieved that we might pass my final day in peace. While Mum and Dad sat outside, I cleaned the inside of the caravan, sweeping up all the sand that we'd brought in from the beach, and I felt so incredibly sad. It had become clearer that Dad was slowly disappearing, and I didn't know what to do, or what would come next.

You'll Never Walk Alone

Alzheimer's can take away all the light in family life and robs you of normality. Even the shape of the word looks like it's going to attack you. It strips you of precious moments and possible memories. As we grappled with this hideous disease, it was as if Dad, Ted McDermott, had lived two lives and was two different people. Night used to be the time that the performer came alive, but it now became the time that we dreaded the most. I also realize that Mum and I struggled alone for a long time – looking back, perhaps we were in denial about what was happening. When he had a good day, it was like being thrown a scrap and it allowed us to pretend that the good outweighed the bad.

It was partially about control, I suppose, and the fear of letting go, because it meant finally admitting that Dad wasn't himself any more. We'd always been a big and loving family and we sorted out our own problems, but even though Dad's brothers and sisters did provide words of support, his care fell to me and Mum. It was hard for Dad's siblings to see their brother standing in front of them but not be able to recognize them. He wasn't the brother who protected them and was prepared to put food in his pockets so they could share in his good fortune – he couldn't even remember their names. I also ended up trying to protect them from the worst of Dad's behaviour and, as time went on, the whole situation dragged me down. Friends would listen to me go on and on and on about the madness up in Blackburn, but I'm not sure they realized the extent of the aggression we were dealing with. I just wanted someone to tell me what to do and then I would do it. John thought that it was time for Dad to go into a home, but I knew deep down that it wouldn't be right for him. He was still there – some part of Dad was still there – and I could only think of the utter terror he would feel if he realized he was being taken away. I couldn't bear that because, despite him still being so abusive, there were also moments of kindness that lulled us into a false sense of security. The uncertainty brought out a whole number of issues in me that I wasn't sure how to process.

When I wasn't in Blackburn dealing with the threats and abuse, I'd be down in London worrying about it all. But drowning is a quiet event – I covered up the struggle for air with partying down in London whenever I could, to the detriment of my relationship with John. I was completely adrift. I felt like I was living in a constant anxiety attack, dreading every text message or phone call, waiting for the next one to wash over me – because often it signalled another drama back up north. I was travelling to Blackburn from London every second weekend because I was so worried about Mum's safety.

You couldn't even keep a door closed in the house – if Dad came across one, he would karate-kick it open, including the bathroom door. We would hardly sleep as he would be pacing around the house in the middle of the night, muttering abuse. It was quite clear that he no longer knew who I was, no matter how many times I told him, and he would fly off the handle if I even spoke a word to Mum. We were living in a war zone.

One dreadful weekend in August 2015, it got so bad that, when I went up to stay, I would often put my suitcase against the door in the spare room – just in case Dad came into the room. His behaviour was so erratic that I was terrified. Sometimes he would burst in, hit me and start calling me a toerag, while other times he'd be there but quiet, and I'd wake up startled and we'd both frighten the life out of each other.

'Bloody hell, Sime! I thought you were someone else.'

It got to a point where we really couldn't cope with the aggression and abuse any longer, so after reading advice on Talking Point – the Alzheimer's Society's online forum – I called the social services helpline. Unfortunately there was no one around to come to visit us until the Monday. We were told the only options were to try and keep Dad calm until then, or call the police – which may have meant he would be sectioned and taken away for our safety – something I really didn't want to happen. On the Monday I called work, explaining that I would have to take more days off because of what was going on at home. I was so worried about Mum – I didn't want to leave her in the house alone with Dad.

The doctor had arranged to come to the house with the social worker. I wrote a detailed list of things I needed to talk to them about when they arrived. It was a rainy Monday and Dad was sitting in the back room fuming about something while I waited in the front room until I could see them walking down the road. I dashed out and pulled them to the side behind a bush – I was worried Dad would see that I was talking to them. We talked about his condition and what had gone on that weekend. I started going through the list of what was happening at home and by the time I got to the third point, I realized how utterly terrible things were. My voice began to break. I couldn't understand how we had got to this point. In the end, I just handed over the list, as I knew if I tried to read out another point I would completely break down.

'Don't worry – we'll sort it,' said the woman from social services.

'Whatever you do, please don't ask him anything about his memory,' I begged. 'It will just upset him and we'll have to deal with the consequences of that all day.'

Dad was still in complete denial. He insisted that it was everyone else who had problems and that he was just fine. We were accused of stealing his money, lying to him, hiding his wallet, talking about him behind his back and even trying to poison him. Everything he said to us was either abuse or a threat about how he was going to either break our legs or throw us into a canal.

I brought them both in.

'Hello, Eddie! We're just doing a home check on you and Linda to make sure that you're both looking after each other,' the social worker said. 'Can we ask you a few questions?'

Dad's face was like thunder. 'You can do. But I might not answer them.'

'Dad, they're only here to help make sure you and Mum are healthy,' I said.

'There's nothing wrong with me. It's her who needs her head checking,' he snapped.

Dad was sitting in his usual armchair while Mum made some tea for everyone. The doctor pretended to do a body examination on him, checking his knees and pulse.

'So, Mr McDermott, how do you think your memory is?'

I nearly fell off my chair. It's only now that I realize that he had to ask that so that he could see Dad's reaction.

'Top hole,' Dad snapped. 'It's these you should worry about,' he added, pointing to me and Mum.

But I could tell from Dad's eyes that he was petrified about what was going on. It was a mixture of anger, sadness and confusion and it was horrible to watch. As he looked at me I could see the fear in his eyes – but I could also see the anger – as if to say, 'Why have you done this?' Dad was at his most fragile, even though I knew he was ready to kill us. After a while the social worker asked if Dad would take her out to see the garden so that Mum could talk directly to the doctor. It was hard for Mum to be honest about how bad things were and she spent a while being diplomatic and skirting around the reality of how hard life had become. I knew she felt like she was betraying Dad, but after some prompting, she opened up.

One of the main issues was that Dad was refusing to take his medication, so the first thing was to change it to liquid form, which could be given more easily. Then it was arranged that the social worker would come to the house every Wednesday to keep an eye on things, just in case Dad's behaviour changed dramatically. That lasted two weeks as Mum felt that the social worker coming round was interfering with their routine. This is something that was to become a source of many disagreements between us in the future.

It was a traumatic time but I had to return to London to get back to work. As I came down the stairs with my bags, Dad turned to me and said, 'Why are you wearing women's clothes?'

I couldn't believe it. Was he joking? Was he confused? Did I dress like a girl? My head was all over the place.

As I got into the taxi to take me to the railway station, the driver turned to me and said, in a broad Indian accent: 'Do you like music, mate?'

Before I had the chance to answer he switched on the CD player and played 'Sugar, Sugar' by The Archies. It was a total paradox. We drove through Blackburn as he sang along in broken English while I sat there next to him, tears streaming down my face. We arrived at the station and I paid him the fare. As I got out of the car, he called me back: 'Mate, look after yourself. You'll get through this.'

I was wiped out and I cannot describe how utterly alone I felt when I returned to my flat. I really didn't think I could face another day, let alone another week, of the chaos. I'd seen the number for the Alzheimer's Helpline lots of times but never thought about calling it – that was for other people. I wanted to phone my friends Nick or

Felipe to talk about what was going on at home, but I didn't feel I could do it again as they'd heard it a million times. I just wanted it all to end. It sounds horrible to say, but I wanted Dad to disappear and then our lives would be better. We were all in a very, very dark place.

I picked up the phone, dialled the number, and a woman answered.

'Can I help you?' she said.

'It's about my dad…' I started, and I completely broke down.

It was exactly the same sort of crying that had happened when Dad said that I was a failure. I could hardly talk and each time I tried to get anything out I would start to cry again. This illness had finally beaten me and I felt there was nothing left I could give. I hadn't got a clue about what I was doing or what I was supposed to do. How long was it going to go on for? I felt like I was living in hell. Through broken sobs, I told the woman on the end of the phone what was going on. To say I was depressed would be an understatement.

'I don't think I can do this any more,' I said, describing Dad's aggression. She let me rant on about him, just listening, understanding.

'You can do it and you are doing it,' she said. 'Your dad would be proud of you both.'

The woman continued to listen as I talked through everything that had happened in the last few years. She explained to me what Dad was going through – how all his aggression and anger was just his fear coming out. In all this madness, I'd struggled to think of it from Dad's point of view before; I'd only seen his behaviour and how it was affecting us. I didn't for one moment consider what was making him behave like this, what was triggering it, what caused these rages. Dad was frightened and alone and it must have been as terrifying for him as it had been for us. I had to put myself in his shoes and try and see things from his point of view. That conversation changed the world for me. I really was at my lowest point, but that anonymous woman at the end of a phone line lifted me up and gave me the courage to carry on. I had no idea what I was doing and I felt alone, but that was nothing to what Dad was going through. I wasn't going to give up – Dad was still there inside, there were still good days when he would remember who I was. I couldn't let him go just yet. When I got off the phone, I said a prayer to myself. I hadn't prayed in years, let alone to an imaginary being up in the sky. 'Please God, let us get through this…' Then I picked up a fork, pricked the plastic on top of a ready meal and put it in the microwave for my tea.

Later that night I called up Mum to see how things were. She sounded upset and as though she'd been crying.

'What's the matter?'

'Nothing,' she said.

'Something's the matter – I can tell by your voice. Has he hit you?'

'No…' Her voice began to falter.

'Well, what's going on?'

'I can't tell you, because if I do I won't be able to stop crying,' she said – and then she completely broke down.

She explained that after I'd left, she'd gone upstairs to have a nap and get away from him. When she woke about an hour later, she went downstairs and into the front room. There she found Dad, sobbing in the dark with a handkerchief covering his face.

'What's the matter, Eddie?'

'I don't know what's going on. Something's not right,' he said. 'I know I'm upsetting people but I don't know why. I don't know why I'm making people sad.'

Mum went to sit next to him on the sofa.

'And I know this is wrong and doesn't make sense but your mum came in here and told me not to worry and that it was just a phase I was going through, and everything would be OK… And I know that's not right because she's dead,' Dad sobbed. 'And then after that my mum came in. And she said the same thing and that I shouldn't worry as people would look after me. And I know it's not right because they're both dead.'

So they just sat there together in silence, on the front-room sofa, hugging each other and crying their eyes out. As Mum told me this down the phone I was crying, too. It was heartbreaking. My poor Dad. This raging monster that had been with us for the past few years was as frightened as anyone. We couldn't let him walk down this path alone.

For the next few months, things were very much the same. Mum and Dad would go to St Stephen's most Saturdays so Dad could sing and I'd go up every couple of weeks or so. He would still have his rages and we would be walking on eggshells, but there was more sadness in Dad. One time Mum was washing up in the kitchen and Dad couldn't find her; later, she found him upstairs in their bedroom crying. He thought she'd walked out and left him and he was all alone.

One weekend, Mum and Dad came to visit me in London. As soon as Mum arrived I could see on her face that she was exhausted and needed a break. Dad had a face on him and I was dreading what the weekend would bring.

'Come on, Dad, let's go for a walk.'

Initially he was a bit wary about leaving the flat without Mum, but I eventually managed to persuade him to come with me and give her some peace. It was a Thursday evening and there were loads of office workers around having after-work drinks. Dad was chatting away about everything and nothing. Most of the time I switched off as a lot of the things he said were either made up or confused monologues. It was a mild spring evening and I took him for a walk through Borough, down the High Street, and along the South Bank.

I was desperately trying to find a pub that wasn't too packed or full of loud drunken men in suits. I just knew that they wouldn't understand Dad's condition and it would turn into a pantomime.

Eventually we came to The Union Jack, a pub a few streets back from the Tate Modern. I found us a seat and went to the bar to order some drinks. The barman had long black hair. As I was waiting Dad suddenly appeared next to me.

'You've got beautiful hair,' Dad said to the barman.

The barman looked confused. 'Sorry, mate?'

'Dad!' I tried to shut Dad up before he said anything else.

'What's the matter with you? She's beautiful!' Dad exclaimed to me.

The barman looked furious. It looked like my dad was flirting with him, which essentially he was. It was bonkers.

I tried to distract Dad away from the bar but he turned back to the barman, laughing and pointing at me: 'Look at him. He's scared of talking to beautiful women like you!'

The barman stood open-mouthed. I was burning with embarrassment. 'I'm sorry. He thinks you're a woman,' I said, making things ten times worse. As we walked to our table, the rest of the bar was in hysterics.

'So, where are you from?' he said, sitting down.

'Blackburn.'

'No – but where do you live?'

'I live in London, Dad – where we are now,' I said.

'Oh. My son lives in London. Yeah, he lives near London Bridge. Do you know him?'

Although part of me knew Dad would forget who I was most of the time, he'd never spoken to me directly like this as though I was a stranger. This was new territory and I didn't know what to say.

'Do you know him?' he asked again. 'He's called Simon.'

'Urm… urm, no. I may do,' I stuttered, not knowing what to say.

'He's from Blackburn as well. Where do you work?'

'Barnardo's.'

'You're kidding me! You work at Dr Barnardo's? Just wait until I tell Linda. Our Sime lives in London AND works at Barnardo's!'

I had no idea where this was going but I just had to go along with it.

'You might know him. Everyone thinks he's a bit soft, but he knows what's going on.'

'What do you mean?' I said, but in reality I was thinking, 'What? SOFT!'

'Well, he's not like a normal bloke. Not like me and you. I don't know what's going on with him. But he's OK. He knows a few people in London and they like him. He works at Dr Barnardo's. He's a writer. With computers. He's got my looks, but he's more like his mother.'

Everything was all jumbled up. There were bits of truths mashed together with whatever was going on in his brain.

'What's Linda like?'

'Well, you know. Linda thinks a lot about things before she does anything. She's got her head screwed on. He's like her. I'll just jump into things and not think.' He paused and sipped his pint. 'No, Linda knows what she's doing. She takes forever to make a decision but once she makes it, her mind's set on it. I let her sort out everything. I wouldn't know what to do without her – she's a diamond.'

'Where did you meet?'

'Oh, I met her at Blackpool one New Year. I was working up there, sorting out the entertainments. I was walking through these revolving doors and she was on the opposite side and I knew that one was for me.'

I sat there in silence with tears pouring down my face as he talked about his life with Mum and his son. He was so proud of me and he was so much in love with Mum. It's something I'd never ever heard Dad say my entire life. I thought he didn't care, but here he was, describing his son, me, in every detail with so much pride in his voice. I sat right in front of him, listening to him tell the story of his life, and he had no idea who I was.

He talked to me about how he would always wind his son up.

'When he was growing up and going on about this and that, I'd always say the opposite,' he laughed.

'Why was that?'

'He wouldn't learn otherwise...'

I took a huge gulp of air. All those arguments where I would storm out, all those doors being slammed. I just never knew why he had to be so difficult; I didn't think Dad got me. But of course he got me, he understood me completely, and even with all my flaws and failings, I made him the proudest man on the planet. And at that moment, that was all I ever really needed to know.

We finished our drinks and made our way out through a side room that had been roped off for a private meeting.

'I'll give you a song,' Dad shouted as we pushed through the confused crowd.

'I'm sorry, this is a private event. You need to leave.'

'It's OK, we're just passing through,' I said. 'We can't get out the other way.'

'Name a song and I'll sing it,' Dad said.

'EXCUSE ME. Do you mind leaving, please?' one woman bellowed at us.

'Go on, Mrs!' said Dad, oblivious to where we were. 'Name a song and I'll sing it! Go on!'

'This is a private event, thank you,' the woman snapped.

'Come on, Dad,' I said and put my arm around him. He tripped a few times over some bags and chairs, but eventually we got out and walked back to my flat, where Mum was watching the TV. Dad went off into the other room.

'Everything OK?' she asked.

'Yeah.'

'What's the matter? You look like you're about to cry. Has he upset you?'

'No. Not at all. Really, not at all,' I said.

After Dad had finished, I went into the bathroom. Mum was right – I did feel like crying. I felt so incredibly sorry for him – he was fading away and I didn't want any more of him to disappear.

Singing In the Rain

By spring 2016 the music was back and firmly a part of Dad's everyday routine. Every weekend I came up, he had his music on downstairs in the back room, where we had set up his record player. One day I was listening outside the door as he belted out 'Mack the Knife' – when all of a sudden, he got all the words mixed up. He tried to get back into the song, but the words were all jumbled. Usually if he forgot lyrics he'd cover them up with something similar and would be able to get away with it, but this was a major mix-up. Just a load of random words that had nothing at all to do with the song. It was a sobering moment, to think that, at some point in the future, this would be the norm and I'd never be able to hear my dad sing like he used to. Then I imagined the house silent – with no music or no sound of Dad's voice. Despite how embarrassed I'd been of his singing when I was younger, I knew his voice was everything to all of us; it was who he was. I wondered if he knew he'd mixed up all the words and how he felt as he tried to sing this song that held so many memories for him. 'Mack the Knife' was Dad's song – his signature tune – but now he had begun to forget the words that he'd sung hundreds of times before.

I realized that we had to try and capture Dad's voice while we still could. That last Christmas, I decided that, as his present, I would take him to a studio and record him singing. I knew that time was running out and we had to do something quickly if I wanted to be able to play

his music in the future. I set about doing some research and narrowed
it down to three places. I called and explained about Dad's condition
and that there might be some aggression to deal with. The first two
studios said they didn't feel comfortable with that and by the time I
phoned the third place I was thinking about giving up completely.
Thankfully, I spoke to a guy called Seamus from the Shamrock
Recording Studio in Blackburn. I told him the entire situation: 'My
dad's a former club singer – he's about 80.'

'What's he like? Frank Sinatra, Al Martino?'

'Yes! Sinatra, Al Martino, he knows loads, but he's a Sinatra man at
heart. I need to tell you that he's got Alzheimer's and he usually kicks
off at the slightest thing. I just want you to know because it could be
quite a difficult session,' I said.

'Not a problem, don't worry. Which days are you thinking?'

I gave a list of dates and booked something in. Finally we could
make some good memories.

I pulled together some of Dad's old backing tracks and edited them
down, cutting the tracks into the different songs. I had no idea what
was on these minidiscs as I sat down to listen but was happy to hear
that all the usual favourites were there: 'Here in My Heart', 'I Won't
Send Roses', 'Lonely is a Man Without Love'.

A few weeks later, I went back up and played the tracks through
to Dad. His face lit up.

'This is all the stuff I sing.'

'I know, Dad.'

He wanted to play them all day on a loop and I couldn't help but
hope that, just maybe, he was escaping to a better time, far away from
the worry of not remembering. I was excited about the recording and
knew his brothers and sisters would be too – Dad's voice had been
at the heart of the family for years and now we would all be able to
listen to it whenever we wanted to. But on the day of the recording,

he woke up in a terrible mood. You could just tell it was going to be a nightmare of a day.

'Just see how it goes, Simon. If it doesn't work out, at least we tried,' Mum said, trying to reassure me.

His face at breakfast was like thunder and I didn't dare speak as he would just tut and shake his head whenever we opened our mouths. He wouldn't accept any food that my mum touched or tea that she poured, saying that she was trying to poison him.

Getting him to put on a different pair of trousers was impossible. In fact, the simple act of changing his musty trousers meant that Mum and I were both subjected to an hour of abuse. As I watched him ranting about his clothes, I couldn't help but remember all the times I'd watch him get ready for shows and how much of a fuss he would make about the way he looked. Now he hardly ever changed his clothes at all. Worse still, at night, he had started to hide them under his pillow so that Mum didn't even have the chance to wash them. Long gone were the days he would press a crease down the front of his trousers; now they were more likely to be found scrunched up in a ball, hidden away.

Finally, we managed to get in the car. We had told Dad we were taking him to the house of a friend who was going to record his voice, but it didn't really register. 'I'm a professional singer, I don't sing for nothing,' he'd say.

'Dad, we should be paying him, because he's doing us a favour.' I didn't dare tell him that we were paying someone to record him sing.

'I DON'T CARE – as long as they PAY ME,' he snapped. It was a far cry from the man who would happily sing for free.

There was no point trying to explain, it was easier to go with it when things were like this.

However, as soon as we arrived at Seamus's, the showman soon came out.

'Dad, this is Seamus. He's a friend of mine and he's going to record you singing today.'

'Bonjour, monsieur!' said Dad enthusiastically.

Seamus was Blackburn born and bred, over six feet tall, and he towered above us all.

'Right, then. I'm painting the studio at the moment, so we're going to record it today in what is, essentially, the loft,' he said.

'Oh, Christ! What have I done?' I thought. 'This is going to be a DISASTER.'

We all headed upstairs. Dad marched ahead while Mum followed behind, carrying a blue plastic bag full of old CDs, music, a bottle of water and some lyrics to some songs she'd printed off in case she needed to prompt him. Seamus took us into the attic and explained where Dad should direct his voice and which headphones matched up to which mic.

'Nope, nope! I'm not putting anything on my head. My hair will get messed up and I'm a PROFESSIONAL.'

'But, Dad, you won't hear the music if you don't put the headphones on.'

'I DON'T CARE. I GET WHERE I'M GOING AND I'M NOT PUTTING THOSE THINGS ON MY HEAD!'

'Dad, look – I've got them on and I can hear all the music. Just have a try and see if you can hear it, too.'

It went like this for about ten minutes before he eventually agreed to have them on his head.

I walked back into the mixing room and told Seamus we'd go through the songs on the CD and see how it went.

We started off with 'Beyond the Sea'.

All of a sudden, mid-flow, Seamus stopped the track.

'WHAT THE BLOODY HELL IS HAPPENING? THEY'VE STOPPED THE MUSIC. I'M THE SINGER! WHERE'S IT GONE?'

This. Was. A. Nightmare.

'Hello, Eddie – let's go back a few bars and just re-record that bit again,' Seamus said down the line.

'WHAT THE BLOODY HELL ARE THEY DOING? I'M A PROFESSIONAL! I DON'T NEED THESE TWATS TELLING ME WHAT TO DO!' He snatched his headphones off.

I ran back into the mixing studio. 'Hey, Seamus, we can't really restart tracks – he will go berserk. I think the best thing is just to play it through and see what we can do.'

'You're right. My fault, I completely forgot. Normally we'd go back and re-record things.'

'No worries – I'll go back in,' I said and dashed back down the corridor to the recording room.

'OK, Seamus – we're ready now,' I shouted down into the mic.

The music started.

'Linda, what song's this?'

' "Beyond the Sea".'

'I can't stand that song. I usually play with a big band in St Stephen's, they all mob me there.'

I started to worry that this was actually too traumatic for Dad, as if he was stuck between two worlds, but only half in each. He must have felt like his life had been turned inside out and he didn't belong anywhere at all. In his head, he was still a superstar, but the illness had taken away all his charm and made him the absolute opposite. Gone was the quietly confident young lad, who'd do anything for anyone. Now he was just an aggressive, arrogant nightmare.

'Eddie, Simon bought you this for a present and we're recording you so we can give a CD to all your brothers and sisters,' Mum said.

'Oh, OK then. Right, play the music.'

'You'll need to put the headphones on.'

'I AM A PROFESSIONAL. I'M NOT WEARING THOSE.'

I walked out of the recording room and into the mixing room.

'I'm so sorry,' I said to Seamus. 'This is a big mistake. I'll go back in and see if I can get him to wear the headphones and then see what happens – I'll shout when he's ready.'

'Dad, look, if I put these on my head I can hear the band playing.'

'Can you?'

'Yes, look… Why don't you try it?'

'So I put them on my head and I can hear them play?'

'Yes.' I was praying Seamus would take his cue from what I'd said.

'Oh, OK.'

There was a pause.

'WOW, that's amazing! Linda, listen to this. Put this on your head and you can hear the orchestra.'

'I know, I've already got them on,' Mum said.

'What? I can't hear you. What did she say? I can't hear you. Shussh, I'm trying to listen to the music.'

Then he turned towards the wall smiling and shouted: 'Brilliant, boys! Best music I've heard in years.'

He went to the mic and started to sing, but just as the magic began to flow, he kicked off again and we were back to square one.

I was so embarrassed and started apologizing to Seamus over the mic for wasting his time.

'He had it. If he would have just continued…'

'OK. Look, let's give it one more go and if it doesn't work this time, I'll call it a day.'

'Dad, if you put these on your head you'll be able to hear the music.'

'Oh, can you? Brilliant!'

'Eddie, we're going to play "Beyond the Sea" so you just sing along when you want.'

'OK, boss!'

The music started. By now, I had my head in my hands. We were about one hour into the session and I was pouring with sweat, just thinking about all the money I was wasting.

But suddenly he managed the first verse and then the second. 'He's got a brilliant voice,' Seamus said. All I could focus on was the old tape machine that Seamus had going round and round and kept praying, 'Please get through to the end.'

Finally, BOOM! He'd done it.

'Brilliant,' I thought.

The next song kicked in.

'Let's just keep him going as far as he can go,' said Seamus.

Dad nailed every song that we played. There were a few places where he forgot the words, but he was having the time of his life. 'What's next?' he shouted down the mic. The showman was back and finally we had a recording of his voice.

'Top-class professionals,' he kept shouting over his shoulder, thinking there was a band behind him.

We did about fifteen songs non-stop in the first session and Dad was full of praise afterwards: 'Brilliant musicians you've got there. What's your name? Seamus. Brilliant musicians. You should come to St Stephen's one night and I'll get you a gig. Top-class musicians they have on there. They'd love you…'

A week or so later, Seamus sent me the edited recordings and they weren't bad – there were a lot of little mistakes, but they were more or less there and I started to feel more positive about booking another session, especially as Dad's eightieth birthday was approaching. I knew that time was running out with Dad and that things were changing rapidly, and I wanted to put on one last big party for him and the family – it could be our last chance. I thought about how to recreate a night where Dad could sing to everyone. How about bringing back the Eddie Carter Show? 'It's a big risk,' said Mum. 'But we should try it.' When I spoke to the family and friends, however, they were concerned:

'Simon, remember your dad is ill. This could be really stressful for him. Why not arrange a nice meal for him on his birthday instead?'

Maybe they were right. I went back and forth debating whether or not we should do it, until finally deciding: it was now or never – I had nothing to lose.

I booked the upstairs room at St Stephen's and started thinking about the theme. Then I realized – if we were recording him singing, why not turn it into a fake album launch party? I wanted to give something back to the Alzheimer's Society for the way they'd helped me the year before, and decided that we would use Dad's birthday to fundraise too. I'd only called the helpline a few times but it had saved me and shown me that we weren't alone, and that we could support Dad. I couldn't forget how many nights I'd spent trawling through their forums looking for advice on how to deal with Dad's condition. In the darkest of days and nights, they were a lifeline. I thought it would be a nice idea if anyone who donated to the collection on the night received a copy of Dad's CD.

The invitation went out: 'The Teddy Mac 80th Birthday and Album Launch Party'. It was either going to be a huge success or a massive failure – that's if Dad even decided to come on the night. He was still going through a phase of saying at the last minute that he didn't want to go out, leaving Mum all dressed up with nowhere to go and often would be physically threatening if she begged him. Even if they did make it out, he could ruin things by getting jealous and causing a scene, something that was mildly acceptable when they were younger, but now just frightening because of the extent of his vitriol. I hoped that, because they were still going to St Stephen's most weeks, the fact that it was familiar would mean he was more likely to go and that he would feel safe on the night.

Back in London, I started to download all of the songs that Dad used to sing in the clubs and searched for all the lyrics online. If Dad was going to get up and sing at his party, I wanted to make sure that if he did forget any of the words, I could dash up onstage and sing along with him, so that he wouldn't be up there on his own, confused in front of all the family. The last thing I wanted was for him to feel humiliated, especially as it could be his last time performing onstage.

Each day, I listened to the tracks and learned the lyrics as I sat on the Tube travelling to and from work. They were all the songs that I had grown up with, but when the lyrics were there in front of me, I suddenly saw their true meanings. All these stories about love, life and broken hearts. I was still feeling the after-effects of a break-up and instead of these songs being twee and old-fashioned, they became relevant, meaningful and now. 'Songs are just love poems set to music,' Dad used to tell me as I was growing up. I never paid much attention to him when he'd say that. But thirty years later, I found myself sitting on the Central Line in rush hour, hurtling towards Barkingside, trying to hold back tears from pouring down my face as I'd listen to sixty-year-old love songs from Al Martino and Nat King Cole.

In the evening, I'd return to my flat and spend hours going deeper down Internet rabbit holes, listening to Dad's favourite tracks, reading about how they came about, translating the Italian lyrics and discovering the stories behind them. I took them all back to Blackburn and sat on the sofa next to Dad, playing them through my mobile phone. We sat in silence listening to them all.

'This is a great one,' said Dad as we listened to 'I Won't Send Roses'. 'But the reprise at the end is the best.'

'YES!' I said. 'I think so too!'

We had connected – we weren't so dissimilar after all.

By the start of June, I'd collected more of Dad's backing tracks and organized them according to which ones I knew he could sing all the way through and eventually narrowed it down to fifteen. Me, Mum and Dad went back to Seamus's and Dad was on great form. We ran through the tracks in no time. Afterwards we all went for a drive around the Ribble Valley and I put on the music we'd just finished recording. Dad was singing along without a care in the world. I hadn't seen him this happy in months. As we reached Whalley, 'Quando, Quando, Quando' came on. It was a song that Dad always performed, so we all knew the words and began to sing along. 'Play it again!' he said. We must have sung it four or five times non-stop. By the time we got near the top of the hill, Dad was singing away and Mum and I were in the front, laughing at his complete change in personality. I wanted to record it. We'd had such a bad few months and this was a rare moment of happiness worth catching. We had the windows down, the music was on full blast and we were now on to our sixth rendition of 'Quando'.

I balanced the mobile on the front of the dashboard and pressed record.

'Now!' he said, telling us when to start.

It was such a happy moment that behind my sunglasses my eyes were streaming with tears. Out of all this darkness, there was finally this brief feeling of light and normality. Everything had lifted, even the countryside around us felt like it had suddenly burst into song. I glanced over at Mum and I could tell she felt exactly the same way.

'Brilliant!' he said when we finished. 'We should have recorded that!'

We got back home and Dad was exhausted but in a great mood. In fact, he was ten times happier. That evening we went to St Stephen's and he was like a new man – the frown had gone and the aggression had subsided. It was as if there had been a pressure-cooker release, the music bringing back the relaxed and happy Ted, the life and soul of the party, the kind guy who'd help everyone, the Ted liked by everyone. I uploaded the video of all of us singing to Facebook and went to bed. It was a quiet night and we all slept well, and by the time I'd woken up, I noticed the video had received over forty 'likes' (for me, this was a lot). 'This is joyful,' someone had written.

That afternoon Dad and I drove down to Tesco to pick up some milk and bread for Mum. It was a red-hot day, so again we had the windows down. I brought some of Dad's old CDs with me, thinking we could sing along to them on the way. I also brought a bit of Blu Tack to stop the mobile from falling as I was filming – I knew these moments would be precious one day and I wanted to bank as many as I could.

I put the CD in, pressed play and then pulled out of the drive. I could see the change in Dad immediately. The first song was 'Let There Be Love' and we drove along singing at the tops of our voices.

We were driving down Cornelian Street singing 'On the Street Where You Live' and there's the line: 'there's nowhere else on earth that I would rather be'. As soon as I sang those words, I stopped singing – right at that moment, there really wasn't anywhere on earth that I would rather be. I was singing with my dad and he was happy. I'd forgotten all about the Alzheimer's, the aggression, the threats and the upset. For that brief instance, everything in the world was OK; singing like this brought Dad real joy. It soon became clear that others felt the same way, because the videos started getting more 'likes' online. So I created a Facebook page, calling it 'The Songaminute Man', after Dad's nickname, and added a link under each video to a JustGiving page where people could donate money to the Alzheimer's Society. If I'm honest it was great to give something back, but the bigger thrill was seeing Dad happy again and being able to show off his voice. I always felt that he missed opportunities and this could be his one last chance to make it big.

One of Those Songs

I set myself a goal of raising £1,000. That seemed like a decent amount to aim for but in no way did I think we could achieve it. I still wasn't sure if it was the right thing to do. Dad was ill and perhaps putting him online for the world to see wasn't the best thing for him. I questioned whether he would want this while he was unwell. But after much debate, I decided that of course this is what he would have wanted. He loved entertaining people – it was who he was. I dared myself to take the chance, uploaded a video and went to the gym. By the time I came out, the page had received thirty 'likes' and two friends had donated. We had about £50 in the space of an hour. More importantly, people had begun to share the videos with their friends – Dad's music was reaching people.

Throughout the next month, every few days I would upload another video of me and Dad singing. By the end of June we had 150 'likes' to the page. And after I posted 'Volare', the 'likes' on the page suddenly jumped to more than 500. By then I knew that I was doing the right thing. We'd raised £500 by this point, and it wasn't just friends donating money but people I didn't even know. Private messages started coming in from people around the world…

'I'm really proud of what you're doing and it's keeping my spirit a little higher. I'm currently sat with my grandma in hospital as she's been

suffering with dementia badly. We play your dad's songs to her. I just want to thank you for being with us at this hard time…'

'My son has autism and never liked music until he saw the videos of your dad singing. You have unlocked a part of him that was hidden for the last seven years…'

'While out shopping I stood next to a lady who was humming "Volare" and we both stood there laughing, talking about your dad. You are bringing happiness to so many people.'

'I had really bad depression the day I saw you and your dad and your video made me instantly happy…'

'I just wanted to say, that even in those moments with uncertainty and no real clarity, your dad is forever proud of you and the son that you have become.'

The next month or so, each time I'd go up to Blackburn I'd take Dad out for a drive and we'd record a few songs. I remember the day he and I recorded 'Quando' vividly. I'd taken him out for another drive around the Ribble Valley. It was a warm day, so the windows were down and we were both singing at the tops of our lungs. When we arrived in Clitheroe, Dad wanted to keep driving around the town centre so people could hear him so we must have done about three or four laps down the main street. I remember we saw a group of lads outside a pub and the fourth time we passed them, they were all cheering. Dad was waving away and singing. I hadn't seen him like this in years; he was back to his fun, confident self. As I pulled into Sainsbury's car park, 'Quando' started again. We parked up and I was about to turn the CD off when Dad shouted, 'Finish it!' and I thought,

'OK then, let's do it...' and I sang as loud as I could. Afterwards we drove back home to Sunnybower and, for the first time in ages, I felt like I'd bonded with him.

Around this time, some of the videos that I had shared on the page had over 2,000 views; it was amazing that people from around the world were enjoying Dad's voice. An old friend from university – Rob, and his wife Roya and family – were visiting from Australia. One Sunday I made the trip up to visit them. I'd posted a video on the page that morning and, while I was on the train, messages began to stream in. I was so engrossed in replying to people and hearing their stories that I completely missed my stop, adding an extra hour to the journey. Something was happening and I couldn't stop thinking about all the messages that were appearing. People were asking for advice, sharing their own stories – it's something I'd never experienced before.

Meanwhile, I was still planning Dad's birthday party, and after getting the tracks from Seamus, I took them down to my friend Nick to edit. He was a piano player and had produced his own music.

We must have drunk buckets of tea and, as we went through the vocals, Nick was impressed. 'Your dad has an amazing voice – to think that he's holding these notes at his age,' he said. Finally, the cuts were ready to send to Seamus so he could print copies. I'd already created the artwork for Dad's party using #Songaminute as the album title (the hashtag I'd used on all the videos) and calling Dad by his old stage name, 'Teddy Mac'. I'd also found an old image of Dad from his Butlin's days. It was completely creased and covered in green felt tip from me scrawling all over it when I was a kid, but it would do just fine with a bit of editing.

By 19 July we had 700 'likes' on the page and had hit our fundraising target of £1,000. It was an incredible feeling. The party was fast approaching and the one thing I couldn't wait to do was show Mum a final version of the CD. Dad wasn't able to say thank you to her, because he would never know what he was thanking her for, but this was a gift to her for all that she had done for him. On the front of the CD were the words: 'To Linda, our rock'. When I gave Mum the CD she read the track list then turned it over. She gasped, holding back tears – 'Oh, Simon! You stupid thing…' – then ran to Dad to show him. 'Look, Eddie, the CD of you singing,' she said. 'Oh yeah,' he said disinterested, hardly looking at it and putting it on the table.

That day, I uploaded the 'Quando, Quando, Quando' video to Facebook. It was my favourite clip of us and I thought it tied in nicely with his birthday. I'd spent the day with a good friend, Felipe, sorting out things for the party that night. I created three huge banners for the room with #Songaminute on them – the letters cut out from old pieces of card, glued on the back of some black wallpaper I'd found. Everything was set. But as soon as I got home I could tell that something was wrong – I found Mum in the kitchen, crying: 'He's not going.'

Upstairs I could hear him throwing things around. 'I KNOW WHERE I PUT THINGS AND SHE KEEPS ON MOVING ALL MY PISSING THINGS. I'M A PROFESSIONAL AND I CAN'T STAND THESE PISSING AMATEURS AROUND ME.' I went upstairs but he was in a fully blown rage. My stomach turned. I'd made a huge mistake and tonight was going to be a nightmare. He was tearing everything out of the wardrobe, refusing to put any clothes on, raging about how he was a professional and he was surrounded by 'PISSING TWATS'. He was horrible.

But then, just as quickly as he'd turned, he calmed down. I distracted him by introducing him to my friend Felipe and managed to persuade him to get into his clean clothes and brush his hair. We reminded him that it was Saturday night, which meant there was a do on at St Stephen's, and he was invited. He slowly calmed down and got into the taxi. I was holding my breath all the way there, just waiting for the next outburst. We got to the venue and parked up, with me explaining what was going to happen. 'Who is going and why are we here?' he kept saying. Eventually Felipe coaxed him inside and got him to his seat; when I saw him sit down at his table I could feel tears in my eyes – it shouldn't be this hard, but it was.

So many people got up to sing and, finally, Dad himself. A couple of times he was out of step with the music, so I got up onstage to join him. I'm not a performer, but I knew I just had to do it. So there we were, singing onstage together – something we'd never done before. I was singing away and knew all the words to the songs that used to make me cringe. I loved it – and so did he.

Dad still had no idea that it was his party, even when we brought out the birthday cake. I managed to gather everyone for a huge group photo, but in the middle of it Dad leant forward, pushing his arm right into the cake. 'The cake!' Mum shouted as the DJ took the photo.

All his candles were lit as we stood around singing 'Happy Birthday' to him. 'Dow cry, Ted!' someone shouted to him. 'Cry? I dow cry!' Dad said. 'I've got seven brothers and six sisters. I don't cry!' I looked around and saw his sister, my Auntie Jane, with tears pouring down her face. 'He had so much pride in his eyes at that moment,' she told me afterwards. 'I can't stop crying each time I think of it.' Dad remembered his family that night and it was amazing to see.

At the end of the night, Gill, Mum and Dad's old next-door neighbour, came up to me in tears. 'You've done an amazing thing. He would be so proud of you,' she said, wiping her eyes. Dad's story seemed to be touching people, and not just those in the room with us. By the next day, his videos had raised £1,500. I had an old friend, Alex, who ran *The Memo* – a tech-news website. That week he ran a story on his site and posted it on his Facebook page. 'This is going to be HUGE,' it said. I didn't think anything of it.

The rest of that week I spent most of my free time replying to the messages that were pouring in. There were so many of them – it gave me huge comfort to know that there were other people out there who knew what we were going through. That Friday was my last day at work before I took a couple of weeks off for a summer holiday. I was in a handover meeting when suddenly my phone began constantly buzzing.

'Someone's popular,' my manager said.

'Si's put some videos of his dad singing online. I think they're going viral,' said my colleague, Ellie.

'Not really – they're being shared a bit. We're raising money for the Alzheimer's Society…'

'A bit?! You've had 100,000 views on one video alone!' she said.

By then the donations had jumped to £10,000 and my phone didn't stop buzzing every few moments with a new notification. It was crazy – £10, £20, £50 at a time.

The next day, I took the train down to Brighton with Nick, for a much-needed day out. I met him at Blackfriar's station at 8.30 a.m. and showed him how many likes I'd had overnight.

'Oh my God, Si! This is going to be massive!' he said.

'No, it won't. It'll be over by Monday,' I replied.

I put my phone on the table in the carriage and we watched while every few seconds it buzzed as another donation came through. By 3 p.m. my phone had died, but the total had jumped by yet another £10,000.

A few days later I got a flight to Spain for a holiday with my friend Brad. The videos were getting more and more views and, by this time, the Alzheimer's Society had been in touch.

When I arrived in Spain I logged into the page and found that the views had jumped massively again. I called Mum and Dad up to check that everything was OK. Every time I'd go away from Blackburn I had a terrible sense of guilt at not being there while they were at home trying to deal with this horrible illness.

'Simon, you need a holiday. Your dad's fine and I can cope – just enjoy yourself. You need a break...' Mum had said when I decided to go.

By nine o'clock the next morning I was lying in bed, feeling worse for wear after a big blow-out the night before, when Brad called.

'SIMON, you're EVERYWHERE.'

I started getting press requests from the BBC, ITV and Sky. This thing had now taken on a life of its own. I thought it would all be over by the following week, so I wanted to take every opportunity that came along. And I was worried about people recognizing Dad in the street and confusing him – Mum would have to cope with it on her own so I decided to come back from the holiday early.

By the time I landed we had raised nearly £30,000 and I'd been contacted by the BBC. They wanted to send someone round to do an interview for that night's show. I was unsure. Things were still very hit-and-miss with Dad. When anyone asked him a question he would give nonsensical answers, and often just go into a long monologue. I had to think about whether it was fair talking about Dad's illness on TV. Also, I didn't want to confuse him and make him wonder who all these people were coming round to the house. But, despite all this, I knew that had he been fully aware he would have told us to go for it, so I did.

That afternoon, Dave Guest, a reporter on *BBC North West Tonight*, had arrived. Dad sang a few songs and then had a quick interview, but it was clear that much of what he was saying was made up: like how he was the son of a millionaire who owned tens of factories in the Black Country!

We didn't watch the report on the news that night because we were worried that it would just confuse Dad. The next morning it was back to reality for Mum and Dad, who had to be up early as they were taking a coach down to the Midlands for Dad's birthday. But he was refusing to put any of his clothes on or let anyone help him. He looked like Worzel Gummidge and was in a foul mood. I dropped them off at Blackburn bus station and said my goodbyes, looking forward to having a few days to myself.

About ten minutes later, just as I was pulling into the drive, Mum telephoned me: 'He hasn't got his teeth in.' I dashed around the house, trying to think where he would have hidden them, but they were nowhere to be found.

I called her back.

'Try under the mattress.'

I searched under all the beds, but had no luck. Then I went downstairs and pulled up the cushions on the sofa – there I found random pieces of clothing that Dad had hidden, as well as his teeth wrapped up in some tissue paper. I delivered them to the station just as Mum and Dad were getting on the coach with seconds to spare. The world might have been interested in our videos, but there were still the day-to-day challenges of living with Alzheimer's to contend with.

That evening I went back to London as I had to return to work the following week. I bought a pizza from Sainsbury's, watched a bit of TV and then went to bed, plugging my phone in to charge overnight.

In the morning I woke up around 8 a.m. and, as usual, the first thing I did was to pick up my phone. I was half asleep but as soon as I saw the number of notifications from Facebook I sat bolt upright. There must have been thousands, if not tens of thousands, of 'likes' on the Facebook video as well as hundreds of donations to the JustGiving page. On top of that I had around 300 friend requests on my personal Facebook page.

'Oh my God!' I said out loud.

I called up Mum straight away.

'Oh, hi! I was just going to call you. I've had about forty friend requests from people I don't know…'

'Don't accept any of them,' I said.

Mum didn't understand how fast the video was going around the Internet. Neither did I really, so I went through all the analytics on the Facebook page trying to work out how it had become so big so fast and had the shock of my life. The video had been grabbed by a news site in the US, and they'd linked to our Facebook page as well as the JustGiving page. It already had 20 million views since it had been posted a day earlier.

I felt my stomach drop and held my hand towards my mouth in utter disbelief. This was much bigger than I had ever imagined.

Then the phone calls and text messages started:

'Simon – that video is all over the Internet!'

'Si – you're ALL OVER my Facebook!'

The videos continued to be shared and at midday, I was in Soho having lunch with Felipe, when the Alzheimer's Society Press Office called: 'We've had a request in from *Good Morning Britain* and *BBC News*, wondering if you'd speak to them today or tomorrow. And can they send a camera crew and reporter to speak to your dad?' 'Christ,' I thought, 'what do I do?'

My first concern was Mum and Dad and them being in Blackburn with no one helping to manage things for them. I felt like I'd massively let them down by exposing them and Dad's illness to everyone, potentially creating more problems.

'Can we just hold back on everything – I need to think about Mum and Dad. Dad's ill and I need to think if I'm doing the right thing.'

I put the phone down and held my head in my hands. 'Fuck!' I said, panicking. Felipe sat there, laughing his head off. I felt totally out of my depth – how was I supposed to do live TV interviews? What if I froze? What would happen to Mum and Dad in all this? How would it affect Dad? What had I done?!

'Si, just remember why you started this in the first place,' Felipe said. 'You wanted people to hear your dad sing and raise money to help other people like you. Just imagine what you could do and how many people you could help.'

It was the wake-up call that I needed and I called the Alzheimer's Society back.

'OK, I'll do it.'

Suddenly a homeless guy stumbled right next to us, pulled out an aerosol can and started getting high on the fumes. 'Man, you could do with some of that,' Felipe laughed.

I was about to throw myself right into the spotlight, just like Dad had done every night when he got up onstage. I was terrified.

Big Time

Walking into the *Good Morning Britain* studio is very much like walking into a different dimension. It's real life, but not as we know it. My heart was pounding and I was trying to stifle a full-blown anxiety attack while being wired up to a microphone and cameras were wheeled around me.

Nothing really prepares you for appearing on live national TV. I was desperate to pick up the glass of water from the table in front of me, but my hands were shaking so much I didn't dare move. I was asked questions; I knew my mouth was opening but whether anything was coming out was another matter. From the corner of my eye I could see a clip playing of Dad and me singing in the car on repeat in the background.

'He's got a great voice,' someone said.

'Brilliant, cheers,' I responded to every compliment.

The next minute I was standing outside on the street alone. What the hell just happened?

Nick calls. 'Si, you looked great. You looked really relaxed!'

'You're joking. I thought I was about to throw up.'

I walked back home to my flat and telephoned my boss asking if I could work from home in the afternoon. But I couldn't concentrate on anything. I was still getting hundreds of messages on my Facebook page and the JustGiving donations were pouring in. That morning we had officially reached £50,000 in donations. By the afternoon the Alzheimer's Society called again. They had more requests from the BBC. Would I be interested in doing some radio shows in the morning from Broadcasting House? I called my boss and asked if it was OK to come in late.

'Definitely, Simon. Go for it! This won't happen again.'

By 4 p.m. I had received requests from news shows across the world – *Time* magazine, *The People's Show* and *The Today Show* in the US, ITV, Channel 5, RTL in Germany, CTV in Canada, and a message from Thames TV saying that there was a TV series that they'd like to chat to me about. When I called up I discovered it was from *Britain's Got Talent* and they'd love to have me and Dad perform.

That was impossible. I couldn't put Dad on live TV – his behaviour was so erratic it was impossible to predict how he would behave. Plus, I didn't want him to be seen as a circus act: the guy with Alzheimer's who can sing. I knew full well he could knock them out if he was having a normal day, but I just couldn't put him in that situation. I had to put his dignity first, no matter what happened.

At 5 p.m. I received an email from *The Ellen Show* in the US, researching features for their next series.

I called up Nick: '*The Ellen Show.*'

'You're kidding me?'

'I've just been on the phone to them.'

'Fuck, Si! This is amazing!'

I then started to get more text messages from friends all around the world.

'Simon – you're on the national news here in Spain!' from a friend in Barcelona.

Then my friend Kasheik messsaged from New York: 'They've just shown your video on ABC.'

I did a quick Google search and saw that the video was now appearing on news sites all over the world: Poland, France, Germany, Spain,

Argentina, Japan, Korea, Australia, Brazil – and not only was the video appearing everywhere but the messages to the page were pouring in.

One of the messages that stood out was from a woman in the Philippines. She was a single mother looking after her own mother who had dementia and was mostly bed-bound. She didn't say anything particularly deep or wise, but just talked about how sometimes she felt so low about it. I thought of this woman, thousands of miles away, who went to her job every day, looked after her mother every day and sometimes felt down because of the illness. But then one day, after going to work, looking after her mother, feeding her family, she saw a video of Dad singing on Facebook, and maybe, just for a minute, she didn't feel so alone.

That night I could hardly sleep. Before I'd gone to bed we had raised £17,000 in just one day, bringing the total to over £70,000. Amazing!

The next morning the car arrived at 6 a.m. to take me to the BBC studios. It was a beautiful clear morning and there was hardly any traffic on the roads. I was being driven down Regent Street, past Oxford Circus, and I could see the church that was just outside the BBC. It sounds ridiculous, but I had a strong sense that Dad was pushing me into all these situations. It felt as though he was in my head saying, 'Right, Sime – hold your head up. Don't be afraid. Don't let them see.' So I pretended that I wasn't nervous at all – probably just like Dad had been when he first stepped onto a stage.

We must have done around fifteen or sixteen interviews that morning for BBC Local Radio stations. It was a whirlwind.

After the interviews one of the producers came down with a lady in her early fifties, who worked in the office. We had just been introduced when she suddenly clasped my hand: 'I just want to say thank you for everything you're doing. You don't know it but you're giving so much hope to other families going through this. I just want to say thank you on behalf of them.'

I didn't know what to say. When I think of it now it feels surreal. Was that really me she was talking to?

When I went into work for my first day back since the video had gone viral, Bernie on reception shouted: 'I've seen your video with your dad. Brilliant!' and gave me the thumbs up. As I rushed up the stairs someone else stopped me. 'Are you Simon? We've all seen the video with your dad…'

As I walked to my seat, everyone started to clap.

I felt myself shrinking into my chair.

Everyone in the team was excited about what was going on. As soon as I sat down my phone started going again. It was BBC Radio 4 wanting to do an interview for *You and Yours* at lunchtime, followed by Sky News wanting a live broadcast.

I quietly booked a meeting room and took the BBC interview in there, then waited for the Sky News van to arrive. As they pulled up behind the office, I prepared myself for a quick interview about Dad and raising money. Instead it turned out to be a ten-minute debate about dementia care in the UK. I was completely unprepared – I knew nothing about dementia care apart from the time it took us to get Dad diagnosed. Then I realized that all of this was beginning to take over my life.

When I got home after work I went through some of the messages that were coming in. One stood out:

'Hi Mac, I'm writing from Decca records. Your family's and your father's story is a powerful one. There's a clear possibility for a successful charity fundraising single/album here and I wonder if we might explore that. Do drop me a line when you have a moment. Alex Van Ingen.'

WOW! This was it, Dad's big opportunity. I took a screenshot and sent it to Nick.

He called back straight away. 'Si, this is amazing. Just think what you said when you started all this. You said you wanted to raise money for Alzheimer's and get your dad a record deal. This is his chance…'

I called Alex as soon as I came off the phone to Nick.

'Oh, hello! It's great to hear from you. How's Ted?'

I told him everything we were going through.

'Listen, it's just a thought at the moment. We wanted to see if you'd be interested in doing a charity record for the Alzheimer's Society. We've worked with the Military Wives before and it worked really well. We'd love to do the same for you and Ted,' he said.

We arranged to meet the following Tuesday at The Grosvenor Hotel in Victoria.

I called Nick straight back, practically dancing around the room. If this came off it would be the icing on the cake: Dad's first single after all these years.

The following day I had interviews with People TV in the States and CTV News in Canada. Both were live.

Afterwards, one of the producers came on the call.

'I just want to say that everyone in the entire team here is completely behind you. Your dad would be so proud,' he said. By now any nerves I'd had about speaking on live TV had gone. It was a ginormous shift for me. Before I would have been terrified at the thought of speaking in front of people in a small meeting at work, and now I didn't blink at the idea of talking to people across the globe. To be honest, it felt like I had recovered all the confidence I'd lost when I was around 16. I just didn't care any more; this was it. It was Dad's last chance.

That evening I went to breathwork meditation. Because I'd been so down in the past year, a friend, David, told me I should try it. I'd never done anything like it before, and I was a bit wary, but I needed something to keep me sane. After my first one-to-one session I was completely sold and I started going to group sessions too. It would drag up memories from years earlier in what I can only liken to an out-of-body experience. It might sound ridiculous, but that evening I felt I was taken to a different plane of consciousness. Our dog Mac came and sat beside me in the room and it was like he'd come to say that everything would be OK. My lips began trembling and I could feel myself starting to go.

I carried on breathing and my mind drifted to Grandad's funeral. I was 24 again and sitting in his armchair in the house he shared with Gladys, reliving the moment I was sat waiting for his coffin to arrive. I was thinking about how I ran upstairs to the bathroom, so the others wouldn't see me cry. The next thing I knew, memories that I hadn't recalled for years were being replayed as if I was actually there. There were Christmases in Cedar Street when I was a kid with Nan and Grandad. The day the house got flooded and all the carpets were taken out on to the street. The arguments between Mum and Dad. Mum sat sobbing on the floor. Dad going out singing and taking his speakers with him. Sitting in the back of the car with Grandad crying after he was told Nan had three months to live. Everything was replayed like a movie.

I told the group what had happened, and felt a huge burden lifting. It was as though all these feelings that had been building up for years had suddenly been released – which was just as well, as things were getting crazy.

I travelled up to Blackburn to see Mum and Dad; they were just getting on with their everyday lives, sheltered from what was going on. But the interest had travelled and I needed to explain to Mum that this was now a big story.

Their Internet wasn't working properly, which was probably a blessing. They would still get the bus into town on a Thursday to go shopping and have lunch at Muffins Cafe in Blackburn town centre. The waitress there – Liz – always made a fuss of Mum and Dad and she knew how to deal with Dad's condition. It was crazy to think that my parents were in their own little world while, internationally, people were going crazy for the videos of Dad singing.

On the Saturday night, I went with Mum and Dad to St Stephen's Club. When Dad got up to sing the compère gave a small speech about how much he had raised for the Alzheimer's Society. As soon as he mentioned the word 'Alzheimer's' I cringed and signalled to him not to mention it. I was so worried about how Dad would react. He was in total denial about his illness and any talk of it would usually send him into meltdown. Luckily, he was so focused on getting up to sing he missed it. The whole room applauded him and he went on to sing 'Quando, Quando, Quando', the star of the night.

On Sunday afternoon, I drove round to the Larkhill flat where Mum's friend Eileen lived. Mum and Dad were there celebrating her birthday and needed picking up. As they came out of the lifts, I checked the JustGiving page: £100,000.

Amazing!

Mum started crying in the back of the car. Dad had no concept of what we'd done or how much money had been raised. 'Why's she crying? Linda, what's the matter?'

'I'm fine. It's just so amazing,' Mum said and wiped her tears away with a tissue.

I put on Dad's music full blast and we drove back home with him singing away at the top of his voice, while Mum sat there with tears streaming down her face. In the space of a few weeks our lives had changed completely.

That night I had to return to London, so Mum dropped me off at Blackburn railway station. A train had just pulled in and people were walking through the underpass towards me. It was pouring down with rain – typical Blackburn weather – and everyone looked downbeat. All of a sudden an Asian guy in traditional dress and a woman in a burka stopped me. 'Oi, mate,' he said, 'are you that guy who sings with his dad?'

I'd never been recognized before.

'Yeah.'

'Mate, let me shake your hand. I can't stop watching those videos,' he said.

I was completely taken aback. By this time people were looking back and smiling to see what was going on.

But the best was yet to come.

When I went to meet Alex from Decca at the hotel in Victoria, I was a bag of nerves. He was tall, thin, very polite and incredibly well spoken. I felt very Blackburn. We chatted about all the songs that Dad could sing, and agreed: if Alex's boss was happy, Dad would release a single with the royalties from the single split between the Alzheimer's Society and Mum and Dad.

I felt reassured when Alex said: 'Don't worry, I've worked with plenty of artists and understand how they can be – and they don't even have Alzheimer's.'

He mentioned getting a live band to sing with Dad.

'Amazing,' I thought – that's exactly what I'd wanted all those months ago when we made Dad's CD in Blackburn.

I went back to my flat in Borough excited, praying that Alex would be able to get his manager to say yes to the project.

At home I called up Mum and Dad straight away. I was buzzing with excitement.

'Mum, it's me. I met with that Decca guy and he's really keen on signing Dad up.'

'That's great. Can I call you back later? We're just eating our pudding.'

'Oh… Oh, OK.'

I couldn't believe it. I'd just called up to tell them the most exciting thing that'd happened for years and they couldn't speak because they're eating their pudding?!

On the Friday I called up Alex to see where things were, but his boss hadn't had a chance to read through his proposal.

'It's not going to happen. I can just sense it. I think they've probably thought about Dad and his illness and they're not that bothered,' I moaned to Nick.

'Si, give it a chance. They can't make decisions overnight.'

***

I was at work when I saw Alex's name flash up on my phone.

'Would your mum and dad be able to come down to London this Friday? I've managed to get a space to record your dad at the studios.'

I wanted to stand up in the office and scream: 'YES!' 'Great,' I said calmly. 'I'll call you in a bit to confirm but I just need to check with them first.'

I put the phone down and tried to carry on working, not telling anyone. I quietly went to the stairs at the back of the building and called Mum.

'Mum, they want to do it. Half of the royalties are going to the Alzheimer's Society and half are going to you and Dad.'

My eyes were watering. I was so excited, but at the back of my mind was a sadness I couldn't ignore, that all this was going on and Dad hadn't got a clue.

Dad came on the phone.

'Dad, you've got a record contract.'

'Oh. Have I?'

'Yes – they want you to come to London this week and sing with a band.'

'Brilliant, Sime. That's brilliant. What do you mean, a record contract?'

I tried to explain but it was no use. I went back to my desk and dropped my colleagues Robyn and Ellie a message.

'Dad's got signed to Decca.'

They both looked up then Robyn came dashing round.

'Si, this is amazing.'

'Don't tell anyone – he's still got to sing yet!'

'I won't. Oh my God, Si. This is mental!'

Ellie couldn't stop taking about it.

'What's going on?!' someone else asked.

By the afternoon the whole floor knew about Dad being signed up with Decca.

So Mum and Dad caught the coach down from Blackburn to London. It was a warm summer night and they were standing outside the station – Dad in his big winter coat, even though the weather was boiling hot.

I took them for a meal at a local restaurant. Dad was in a great mood and I was confident that the next day would go OK.

But as soon as Dad walked into the lounge the next day, I knew it wasn't going to go well. He had woken up in a terrible mood. He always starts bad days being very distant and his eyes go very dark, often with huge pupils. All the fun from the night before had gone and instead he looked like he was about to explode at any minute.

'Not today. Of all the days, not today,' I said to myself.

'You alright, Dad?'

'I'm alright. Always have been, always will be,' he snapped.

I was right: it was going to be a tough day.

'Did you sleep OK?'

'What? Yeah. Where's the bathroom? I can't find anything in this shithole!'

'It's this way, Dad,' I replied, and took him to it.

He slammed the door. Disaster.

I put on some of his backing songs to try and get him in the mood and Dad started singing 'Quando, Quando, Quando'. It sounded absolutely brilliant but you could sense the tension was rising.

I booked a cab to take us to Angel Studios. Dad was talking away in the back and I thought that finally he had calmed down.

'I'm really nervous,' I said to Mum.

'Me too.'

'What do you mean? Has someone upset you?' Dad said.

'Oh no, nothing...'

The Angel Studios is a converted old church in Islington.

'Hi. We're with Decca and we're supposed to be recording today,' I said to a man sitting behind the small desk.

'Yep – it's the main studio just down these steps.'

We slowly walked down a small flight of stairs, pushed open a huge soundproofed door, and – WOW!

The room was massive and there must have been about twenty to thirty musicians setting up. Strings, trumpets, guitar players, the works... I couldn't believe it.

'Oh, my God!' said Mum.

'I wasn't expecting this,' I said.

Dad, meanwhile, was snapping at us to hurry up. 'Come on, come on, come on, people are waiting for me!'

The ego was rising. Christ! I hoped we would be able to get through this.

Alex came walking up to us.

'Hello!'

I gave him a huge excited hug, which suddenly felt inappropriate.

'I thought there'd be about five people. We didn't expect any of this, I'm blown away,' I said.

'Really? I thought I'd emailed you. This is the Guy Barker Big Band – they're some of the best musicians in the country.'

I introduced Alex to Mum and Dad and he took us to the booth overlooking the orchestra.

I could sense Dad's temper was rising. His face looked furious.

'Do you want a cup of tea, Dad?'

'It would be nice to get a decent drink around here.'

Oh, God!

I went to the mixing booth and made teas for us all, chatting to the guys and trying to warn them that I could sense that Dad's mood was changing.

When I went back out into the recording booth, Guy Barker was making his way in. He was great. He introduced himself to Mum and Dad, but you could tell Dad just wasn't interested.

It was so infuriating. Here was a room full of people all willing to make today a success and the only person who wasn't interested was Dad. If only he could understand what was going on.

'Dad, all these people are here to help make your record. They're going to play outside and if you sing into this microphone they'll take a recording.'

'Don't tell me what to do. I've done this for years. I work with some of the best professionals on the planet.'

'OK, Dad – but if you put on these headphones you'll be able to hear the band when they start playing.'

'Nope. I'm not putting those on my head.'

The headphone situation had returned.

'Please, just for one day let this go smoothly,' I was praying.

His face was like thunder.

One of the sound engineers came into the booth to try and adjust his microphone, which was on a stand.

'Nope, nope, nope! I can't sing into that. You seriously want me to sing into that?' and then he did the laugh that meant he was going to explode at any second.

'Listen, I've worked with THE BEST MUSICIANS IN ENGLAND...'

'Dad, we just need you to sing into this microphone so we can record you.'

Meanwhile, a photographer and a videographer were taking pictures of us. Nightmare! I turned to the video guy: 'Please don't film any of this. I can just feel he's about to explode.'

I pulled the sliding door back that separated the band and the recording booth, and shouted over to Guy: 'Can you play something? It might get us in the mood.'

'What do you want us to play?'

'What have you got?'

'"Beyond the Sea"?'

'That'll do!'

The band kicked in. I was taken aback – I'd never been so close to such a big band before, it sounded amazing.

'Where's that music coming from? It's brilliant,' said Dad.

By this time, we'd given up on trying to get him to put the head-phones on his head and decided that if he could hear the basics of the song he should be able to sing along. It wasn't ideal but it was the best we could do.

'Dad, if you sing into this mic we'll take a recording of it.'

'I'm a professional. I've worked in THOUSANDS… THOUSANDS of clubs…'

'I know, Dad, but we just want to record you singing.'

It was so frustrating. I so desperately wanted him to be able to do this – it was his one big chance.

He got one verse into the song, then the brass and the flutes kicked in. Dad had become so used to being accompanied by just a piano player and a drummer in the clubs that this knocked him completely.

'Nope, nope, nope! I can't work with these twats,' he said, and walked away from the microphone.

The whole orchestra could hear Dad's rant through their head-phones. I could see them all looking over, still playing, while he was having one of his tantrums. It was horrendous.

'I've worked with professionals all my life but I've never worked with TWATS like this before.'

The band stopped and I dashed outside the recording room.

'I'm so sorry – can you give us a few minutes?' I asked.

Dad was shouting furiously in the recording booth.

We had a break and then took him onto the main floor of the studio with the band. Again, each time the trumpets kicked in he would stop singing, complaining at the state of the band he was singing with.

It was so frustrating – this was his dream and at any other time in his life he would be blowing the roof off with the band. But not today.

Both Mum and I felt incredibly stressed. We tried different places where Dad could sing. He was so used to performing with an audience that singing into space was completely unnatural for him. At one point we had him stand at the back of the room next to the bass guitar player. I was stood next to him and remember seeing the guitar player's face just willing him to get through the song without kicking off. But it didn't work.

Eventually we tried standing Dad next to Guy Barker at the front of the orchestra. He loved it there – he thought that the orchestra was his audience and was playing up to them. He was slowly coming back again.

We went through a number of songs – 'Quando Quando, Quando', 'You Make Me Feel So Young', 'Beyond the Sea', 'Let There Be Love' – and then decided to take a break before we returned in the afternoon.

But Mum and I felt down. We went to a local pub and ordered some lunch. Dad hadn't a clue what was going on, despite us telling him a thousand times. I began to wonder whether I'd done the right thing, then out of nowhere he said: 'That band was fantastic. Top professionals.' It was so confusing. A minute ago he'd had no idea where he was and now he was talking about the band.

Just as we finished our food, Guy Barker and a couple of the guys from the band came in.

I walked over to Guy and the rest of the group at the bar. 'I'm so sorry about before. He normally wouldn't be so rude to people.'

'It's OK, it went a lot better than we thought it would,' he said.

'Really?'

I was completely taken aback. He then took me aside. 'All the guys are really committed to this. It's amazing what you're doing – we've all seen the videos and it's just wonderful,' he said.

I brought Mum and Dad over and we had some photos. 'Top musicians, these lads are. Brilliant,' Dad kept announcing.

In the afternoon, we went back to the studio to finalize a few of the tracks. Again, Dad refused to put the headphones on. But he finally started to enjoy himself – it was just the rest of us who were exhausted.

'I think that's that, guys. If there's nothing else then we can wrap up,' says Alex.

There was one song that we hadn't done which, for me and Mum, it was essential to record.

'Hold on, there's one song Dad always sings: "Here in My Heart".'

'OK, go ahead then.'

Dad blasted it out.

You could hear a pin drop. I could see Alex and the sound engineer through the glass looking at each other as if to say, 'Wow!'

'Ted, that was spectacular,' said Alex.

Finally, Dad had arrived.

Volare

It had been an amazing day but we were all exhausted. Dad was in his own world and we could sense that the aggression was starting again. We called it a day and went to bed.

The next day Mum, Dad and I took a train to Wednesbury. It was my cousin's wife Mary's fortieth birthday.

As soon as we entered, Dad had a couple of fans that wouldn't leave him alone. He was having a great time, but the tide was about to turn. I was chatting to my cousin when all of a sudden Mum came up to me.

'Simon, can you give me a hand?'

I thought she meant she needed some help carrying something from the bar, but when I followed her over, I saw Dad threatening Uncle Colin to a fight.

'What's going on, Dad?'

'I know their game. If they want a fight they can take it outside,' he said, raising his fists to Colin.

Uncle Colin was trying to calm him down but Dad was just getting more and more irate. We managed to get him outside and into the car.

'Come on, Dad. It's time to go home now and we'll get some tea,' I said, sitting him in the car.

'I'm so sorry you've had to see him like that,' I said and gave Uncle Colin a hug.

For a split second he looked like he was about to cry.

'Don't be daft. He's my brother, I can handle it,' he said.

Dad was smiling and waving away as we drove off, like nothing had happened.

Uncle Colin and Auntie Brenda had been complete rocks since Dad was diagnosed with dementia. They would always make the time to come up to Blackburn and visit Mum and Dad. It could be incredibly lonely for Mum living with Dad and his dementia, and Auntie Brenda and Uncle Colin's visits were a break from the madness.

They were so patient with Dad and his condition, and it was difficult to understand why he would suddenly try to have a fight with Uncle Colin, who always looked out for him.

On Monday I got a call from Alex at Decca.

'Are your mum and dad free this Friday to come to Abbey Road? We'll do the mastering at the studios and some photos for the press.'

To be honest, I was half-expecting Alex to call up and say that he didn't really feel the recording went that well and we'd have to get Dad back in to record. I was taken aback to hear that they had everything they needed.

By Wednesday, Decca had arranged a meeting with me, the Alzheimer's Society's press team, and their own press and media department at their head offices in West Kensington to go through all the tracks that we'd recorded and to talk about Dad's story.

We talked about what songs we could release as a single – narrowing it down to 'You Make Me Feel So Young' and 'Quando, Quando, Quando'.

For me, releasing 'Quando' as Dad's single didn't feel right. It would just make him seem like a novelty act. Luckily, everyone else agreed. It was decided that 'You Make Me Feel So Young' would be the A-side with 'Quando, Quando, Quando' the B-side.

The team wanted to make it public that Dad had been signed up with Decca as soon as possible, with details of how people could pre-order the single before its release. We were all set.

I came out of the meeting, got to the end of the street and called up

Mum straight away. I was buzzing with excitement. Dad was releasing his first single with a major record label. I was on top of the world.

Mum and Dad arrived from Blackburn on Thursday night and we went to the local Lebanese, as we always did.

On the Friday, I thought it would be great to drive Dad around London with him singing along to his own songs. So, I hired a car and we set off around 10 a.m., just after rush hour. There was no plan as to where we were going but we had the music on and Mum and Dad were enjoying just looking out of the window. But as soon as we came close to Buckingham Palace, Dad burst into 'Quando, Quando, Quando'. At one point, just outside the palace, a cab driver in the next lane noticed us and pointed, mouthing, 'Is that him?!' I just nodded back, smiling, and carried on singing.

As we drove down the side of St James's Park we got stuck in some slow-moving traffic just as 'Quando' started to play again.

'Oh no,' I thought.

Despite driving around all morning with the windows down, I really didn't want the attention while we were sat in traffic and there were tourists everywhere.

But it was too late. Dad was already going full blast and by this point he was literally hanging out the window singing along, having the time of his life. I sat staring straight ahead, sensing people looking.

'Oh my God! They're all taking photos,' said Mum.

It was incredibly embarrassing, but, I have to admit, it felt amazing. By this time there must have been a crowd of about twenty people standing in a group, listening to Dad singing. As we inched up the road, the next song that came on was 'You Make Me Feel So Young'. As ever, Dad was going for it. They must have thought we were from the circus.

Eventually the traffic started to move. By this time there were a group of tourists standing at the traffic lights on my side of the car. As we passed them, one of the guys shouted, 'The Songaminute Man!' as we drove off.

'I can't believe that,' Mum said. 'They knew who he was.'

After lunch, we took a cab to Abbey Road Studios. Dad had no idea where we were going or why, but he was in a great mood and excited.

Alex met us at reception with a couple of photographers and a film crew. We did a few snaps on the front of the steps with a mock-up of the sleeve from Dad's single.

Then we made our way down to the zebra crossing, attempting to recreate the famous Beatles' walk. It was like herding cats. Not only was the London traffic having none of it, honking their horns and shouting at us to get out of the way, but Dad had no concept of why we had to stop in the middle of the crossing. Instead he would help other tourists across the road, behaving like a lollipop lady. I think at one point he was even walking arm in arm with a little old woman. Total chaos.

Afterwards we took a taxi down to a pub to grab a bite to eat. We sat at the back and ordered some food but Dad immediately got annoyed because he was sitting in the corner and 'not facing the audience', a group of people eating their dinner. Eventually the guy opposite caught my eye.

'Is it him?' he asked.

'Yep, it is.' I smiled back.

'I knew it!' he said. He turned to the rest of his table, saying, 'That's the Songaminute Man!' Then he took out his phone and showed everyone on his table the video.

Dad immediately started talking to the table as if they were children. 'Hello! What's your names?'

They were all adults. I had no idea what was going on in Dad's mind at this point. At one point he said he could see a band – the hallucinations had started. We finished our food and then went back to my flat in Borough. It had been a good day.

But the next day, I'd been in the gym for about twenty minutes when I got a message on my phone: 'Come home asap. He wants to go.'

Oh, Christ! This was all I needed. I rushed back home to find Dad slamming the doors, trying to get out of the flat. Mum was in my bedroom in floods of tears.

'What the hell's happened?'

'I don't know, he just suddenly got angry,' she said.

'Let me out! Keep me away from THAT WOMAN. I can't stand her.'

'Well, where are you going, Dad?'

'Wednesbury.'

'But why? We're in London and we wanted to spend the time with you.'

He came straight up to me, his face red with rage.

'I have THOUSANDS of women waiting for me in Wednesbury. They're all queuing up to see me at The Cora. I'm getting back.'

'Dad, wait! We're in London and this is my flat.'

'I don't care where we are. Get me out, I want to get the bus.'

'OK – hold on and I'll take you.'

'Keep away from me or I'll chin you.'

This was all I needed.

I let Dad out of the flat and waited a few seconds to follow him.

'Keep away from me, I warn you. I'll chin you.'

'Come on, Dad – let's go for a walk and get a coffee.'

'Why are you following me? You just get back with her and carry on with what you're doing. I'm getting back to Wednesbury.'

'Dad, we're in London.'

'Are we? Right! Well, I'm going back then. This place is deadsville.' And he stormed off.

'Dad, come on. It's me, I'm Simon, your son.'

'I don't care who you are or what you do. Keep away from me or you'll have two broken legs.'

No matter what I said he was having none of it. I let him storm down the street but gave him some distance, watching him working out which way to go. Then he came back up the street, raging and talking away to himself.

Mum and Dad were returning home to Blackburn that afternoon and I was terrified that he wouldn't have calmed down by then.

Watching Dad in this rage while being so lost was horrible to see. Whoever he thought I was at that moment in time, he utterly hated me. And Mum. It was pure rage.

So there we were. Dad storming through the streets of Borough, past tourists going to Borough Market, and disinterested Londoners, telling people to, 'Get out my pissing way' with me dashing after him, apologizing to everyone.

I eventually caught up with him and tried again to reason with him.

'Dad, are you looking for the bus?'

'Yes.'

'Well, why don't we go back to mine and have some tea and I'll take you there afterwards?'

'OK then. But make sure she keeps away from me.'

I got him back to the flat and made a cup of tea.

'There's something wrong with her. She's cracking up. I don't know what it is. I do everything to please her...'

'Maybe she doesn't feel well.'

'Do you think?'

'Why don't you go back in and check that she's OK?'

Mum was still in my bedroom. Her poor face was red from crying. She was wearing some of her best clothes for London, but she looked utterly broken. It was horrible to see.

'Go on. Why don't you ask if she wants some tea?'

'OK then.'

Dad got up from the sofa and went into the bedroom.

'What's the matter with you?' I heard him say.

I let them get on with it. I knew that he was now a lot calmer. His rage had gone and he just wanted to make sure that Mum was OK.

'Are you OK, you two?' They'd been talking calmly for a while and I'd gone to check on them.

Dad had his arms around Mum and they were cuddled up on the bed.

'Do you want a cup of tea?'

'Go on then, Sime. Have you got any cake?'

Things were OK.

But not for me. I felt fed up and drained. I just wanted all this aggression and shouting to end. Who in their right mind would put up with all this drama constantly? I felt that I had nothing to give anyone but stress. I'd go through Facebook and see hundreds of pictures of people on holiday in Mykonos or Ibiza, including my ex, who looked like he was having the time of his life. It just compounded my misery. I felt utterly alone.

I sat on the couch and stared at the wall.

That afternoon, as Mum and Dad were packing their suitcases to go back to Blackburn, Mum came into the lounge.

'What's the matter with you?' Mum said.

'Nothing,' I said and just stared at my phone, scrolling through the Facebook newsfeed.

'What's the matter? You look like you're going to cry.'

'Honestly, it's nothing. I'm just tired. It was busy yesterday.'

'Come on — what's the matter?'

'I'm fed up.' I buried my head in my hands.

She came and sat next to me.

'What's happened? Why are you so upset?'

'It's just everything.'

'What do you mean?'

'It's just everything. I mean, look at us. Look at me. I'm 40. I'm single. And this. All this. Who in their right mind would want anything to do with this?'

'Come on, you've got loads going for you. You're still young. You've got a good sense of humour. You're good-looking. You've got your own flat,' said Mum, reeling off anything positive to try and make me feel better.

'But who would want any of this? No one in their right mind would want to be in a relationship with me with all this…' It felt like everything was falling apart. I'd never be able to introduce a partner to Mum and Dad without the madness getting in the way. If I'm honest, all I wanted right at that moment was to know that there was someone who would be there for me; who knew what it felt like to be in the midst of this madness; who would say, 'I know this is shit, but I'm here for you no matter what.' But there wasn't.

Dad entered the room. 'What's happened?' he said.

'Nothing…'

'Well something's happened. If anyone's done anything to you, I'll chin 'em, Sime!' he said

'Nothing's happened. I'm just tired.'

I ordered a cab and Mum and Dad were whisked off to Victoria Coach Station.

A couple of months earlier I had handed in my notice at work as things were so difficult at home. The plan was to move back to Blackburn for a while and get a temp job while helping out Mum at home with Dad. That was before everything went crazy.

At my last week at work I was stressed out, trying to get my handover notes finished and replying to messages on the Songaminute

Facebook page. There were still hundreds of comments and messages coming in every day, and I was trying to build Dad's website ahead of the press releases going out on Friday. I was up most evenings, trying to sort the website using a painfully slow Internet connection. I was exhausted but knew I had to keep going as this was Dad's one and only chance.

One night I was on the online chat to the web host, trying to solve the problem with the site. Whoever was chatting to me in customer support suddenly stopped.

'I've seen your dad's videos – they're brilliant!' he wrote.

Thursday was my last day working at head office in Barkingside. It was time to say goodbye to the team. By now most people in the building knew that Dad was making a single. People came up to me all that week, revealing that they were going through exactly the same thing as we were. It was incredibly humbling to think that all these people I worked with hadn't mentioned a thing about what was going on in their own home, and yet they'd now decided to share their story with me.

I said my goodbyes and stepped out the door. Then I heard a banging on the windows. The entire team was taking photos and waving at me.

'Are you famous or something?' said a woman as she got out of her car.

'Not at all. My dad is,' I said, and walked off.

As I walked towards Barkingside Tube for the very last time, I got a call from Decca Press Office.

'Simon, can you do a quick interview with *The Times* as soon as you can? It's just for a small news item but they need some quotes.'

'For sure.'

'OK. Everything's ready. The press releases have all been sent out. How's the website looking?'

'Oh, fine. It's going to go live later today.'

I was lying through my teeth. I was having loads of issues with the site's hosting company, and couldn't get the webname to link to the site.

'If you need anything, call me, but everything should be sorted.'

'OK.'

Around 7.30 p.m. I had the phone interview with the guy from *The Times* – it took a lot longer than I'd expected, and I was worried about getting the website up and running.

I worked until late into the night sorting out the site, uploading copy, tagging YouTube videos and making sure all the links were working.

I still hadn't received details from Decca of where people could buy the single. Just as I was going to bed, I saw the messages beginning to arrive on the page.

'Congratulations on getting the record deal! Where can we get the single?' they said.

People had already seen the news. I did a quick Google and found the news was already out on the *Daily Mail*. There was nothing I could do. I just prayed Decca had the links for me first thing in the morning.

That night I hardly slept. I kept waking up to check my phone. The word was out that Dad had been signed by a record company and messages had started to flood on to the page.

By 7 a.m. I was up and showered. My friend Rob WhatsApped me.

'Simes, you're all over the BBC!'

I was too stressed to reply.

At 8.30 a.m. I received a phone call from Decca.

'We've had a great response so far to the press release. How are you for interviews today? We may have a couple lined up for you if you'd like to do them.'

'Yep – no problem.'

'Great. They won't take long, five minutes at most.'

As I left the flat, Nick messaged me: 'Si, have you seen the papers?'

'No.'

'You should! Make sure you get *The Times*.'

I dashed into Sainsbury's on Borough High Street and picked up a copy, expecting a small news item about Dad's single, and turned the front page to find page three devoted entirely to Dad's story.

'Oh, my God!' I said out loud.

I couldn't believe it. Page three! Of *The Times*!

By the time I got back to my flat there was a news crew from Channel 5 waiting at the gates. As soon as they left, BBC News came in. As they were setting up I was doing radio interviews for LBC then Radio 5. It was a conveyor belt of interviews all day. I was excited but exhausted, and had a huge cold sore on my top lip.

Someone from Decca had come round to help organize everything. 'I've never experienced anything like this,' he said. 'This is unprecedented, mate.'

By the afternoon I was going live from my living room to CTV breakfast news in Canada. Then it was an interview with ITV's Nina Nannar, followed by Sky News.

Around 5 p.m. I was being driven to the Channel 5 News studio and I had two live radio interviews, which I did in the car on the way there. I felt like Beyoncé. By this time I had no idea who they were with. It was an utter whirlwind, but I had to keep going. This was Dad's last chance of making it big and no way did I want to miss a thing.

When I arrived at the news studios, the nausea kicked in. I hadn't eaten properly all week and had been up most nights trying to sort the website ahead of the press release going live. I sat down in the green room with the news presenter and the rest of the production crew. Despite the coffee I felt myself getting the sweats – the ones that you get just before you're about to be sick. I couldn't hold it in any longer so I took myself to the bathroom, where I retched up nothing but coffee. Ugh! How was I going to be able to do this?

I went back to the green room and made myself another coffee with four teaspoons of sugar. Everyone was asking questions about Songaminute and Dad. I was in a complete daze. The next minute I was being taken into the studio. It was a quick chat. 'If it wasn't for the Alzheimer's Society and their phoneline, I don't know where we would be,' I said. 'So it's kind of a thank you, to put something back.' And then we were off-air.

I caught a train back to Blackburn that night but missed the 10 o'clock news. Mum and Dad were in the front room having a cup of tea.

'Did you watch it?'

'No, we haven't seen any of it,' Mum said.

In a way I was glad. I didn't want Dad to suddenly see his face all over the TV. He was confused enough as it was and I was scared of doing anything that might confuse him further.

I tried to explain what had happened that day, but Mum didn't really understand how manic it had been with the interviews. They had been out shopping in Blackburn that afternoon, having their usual lunch at Muffins Cafe.

Before bed I went upstairs and searched for the ITV News report on the laptop.

There we all were: the story of how all this had happened. Me and Dad singing in the car. The trip to Abbey Road. Why I'd decided to fundraise for the Alzheimer's Society. All in a two-minute package for the national news. I sat there in silence, wide-eyed.

'My dad's not completely disappeared. He's still there. He's still my dad. He's still inside. He's just a bit jumbled up...'

To think that all this was happening and Dad had no idea. I felt a mixture of pride and guilt. This was Dad's story and he wasn't here to tell it. It shouldn't be me being interviewed – I felt like a con man.

I clicked on to the Channel 5 news report on YouTube.

'When the videos of 80-year-old Ted McDermott singing in the car were posted online they became an Internet hit. Ted, who has Alzheimer's, now barely recognizes his son Simon, but still remembers the words to all his favourite songs,' said the reporter.

Again they showed clips of Dad at Abbey Road signing his single and me and Dad driving around the Ribble Valley singing.

By this time I was sat in the spare room, surrounded by boxes, tears streaming down my face. I felt like I was watching a movie.

'It just makes him happier. When we drive and I look round I can see him smiling. So I'm kind of like – he's happy – and that's the most important thing,' I told the reporter.

The report ended: 'He always dreamed of making it big. Though his memory is fading, Ted McDermott has finally achieved his goal.'

I sat and sobbed at the utter tragedy of it all. Happy-sad tears were pouring down my face as I sat in silence thinking about the last few months. I didn't care how many people bought the single. Even if just one person bought it, the fact would remain that he'd done it. He'd finally made his record. I shut the laptop and went to bed.

Epilogue

'How's your dad?' Carol Vorderman asked me when I got up onstage.

'Yeah he's fine,' I said.

In reality, we'd had a difficult few weeks. After I'd moved back to Blackburn at the start of October, Dad's aggression had reached new heights. Since the clocks had changed and the evenings began to get darker earlier, he would often be up all through the night, taking things out of wardrobes, pulling things out of drawers, slamming doors, switching lights on and off. It was exhausting and, as ever, poor Mum took the brunt of it.

It was back in early September that I was told Dad and I had been nominated for a Pride of Britain Award, but there'd been so much going on (packing my flat, moving up north) that it hadn't really sunk in until Lynn – my cousin's wife – and I walked down the red carpet to Grosvenor House in London. We were surrounded by press, TV cameras, celebrities and fans; it was madness.

The weekend that I left Blackburn to go to the awards, Dad was in a terrible mood. I don't think either Mum or I had slept properly for days. On the morning I left, after telling Dad that I was going to London, he literally threw my suitcase out of the front door, telling me to 'Piss off then. I can't stand you. And take her wi ya!'

Mum was obviously upset by this, so I just said I'd wait outside and call a taxi to stop any further upset. I grabbed my suit holder and sat on the front step with my suitcase waiting for the taxi to arrive. It was November and I was freezing and this was hardly a way to celebrate being invited to the TV event of the year.

On the train down, I just stared blankly out of the window trying to understand why he seemingly hated me so much that morning. To think I was about to go and collect an award for him while all this was going on upset me massively.

Suddenly I got a call from Mum.

'Simon, your dad's here and he wants to speak to you...' she said.

I got up and walked into the vestibule of the carriage so I could speak properly.

'Sime?'

'Dad? Are you OK?'

'Simon? Where you going?'

'London. What you up to?'

'Oh, brilliant. Your mum said you were going away...'

'Yeah, I'm on the train...'

Dad started to laugh nervously.

'I thought you were someone else. I didn't know it was you...' he said, laughing.

I had a finger in one ear as I tried to listen to him. I could tell that he was upset.

'There's something wrong with my head and I get confused some-times. I'm not angry with you. I just... I just thought you were someone else.'

I couldn't believe what I was hearing – it was the first time he'd ever acknowledged that something wasn't right with him.

'Dad, it's OK. Don't worry about it...'

'You know me and your mum are really proud of you. You're our number one and we love you...'

A soon as he said that the tears started. I could hardly speak. Here was a man who an hour earlier was calling me a twat and trying to push me out of the house. Now he was saying I made him proud. It was a rollercoaster of emotions.

'Dad, and I'm really proud of you too. You know I love you...'

'I know you do. Hold on, speak to your mother...'

Mum came on the phone.

'He's been very upset since you've gone. Crying...'

'Oh, Mum, I'm so worried about you both.'

'Don't worry, just have a good time. Say hello to Lynn and Nick and everyone...'

By now Dad and I had raised about £130,000 for the Alzheimer's Society. The money was ring-fenced so that all of it would go to help fund the National Dementia Helpline to help other people like us. Whenever I'd take Dad out to Tesco, he'd get recognized. He loved talking to people, so would happily chat away for ages. After one visit, about six or seven people must have come up to speak to us. As I drove him out of the Tesco car park afterwards, he turned to me and said: 'Well, I knew I was popular, Sime, but I didn't think I was *that* popular...'

I felt like a millionaire. If only he could really understand what had happened in the preceding weeks.

The single reached Number 3 in the iTunes charts, but when they included the streamed plays, it pushed us right down to Number 43 in the official charts. We decided to launch a crowdfunding campaign to make Dad's album, with people paying £12.99 in advance to help fund its creation, and in return they'd receive the CD. After a few months of crowdfunding, the Guy Barker Big Band re-recorded some of Dad's backing tracks and they sound amazing. It still doesn't feel real, especially when I think about those dark, dark days just a few months before.

I was still worried about how much we should expose Dad to some of the reports on TV. But he ended up watching the *Pride of Britain* show, excitedly saying to Mum: 'That looks like our Sime.' He'd forgotten about it ten minutes later though. Now and again he does introduce me to Mum as the person who made him Britain's Number One Singer. (A title that was given to him by the Queen, apparently.)

One night we also let Dad listen to himself on the *Clare Teal* show on BBC Radio 2. It was a chat about his story as well as playing some of his favourite songs. I will never forget that night. Mum had made some tea and we were all sat in the front room with Dad sat next to me. As he listened you could see the realization sink in. 'That's me they're talking about! That's me!'

I was glowing inside.

'We've got to get to London!' he announced.

Dad would also regularly tell people about his trip to London where he sang with an orchestra. But it's very mixed up. He would often tell the story about how he got off a bus in London, turned right, went down some steps, sang into a machine in the wall, typed in a number and out came 'WADS OF MONEY'. 'Just for singing!' he exclaims. If only this were true. Instead he fused together going to a cash machine with recording his single with the orchestra. 'Next time you go to London, Sime, make sure you look out for that machine!' he would tell me.

We have received thousands of messages from all across the world – giving advice, sharing stories or just asking how we all are. It's been incredibly humbling to think that people have taken the time out of their day to make contact. And when I mean thousands, I mean thousands – it's been impossible to reply to everyone. But those stories, crossing each other from different corners of the planet, broke down the walls of our prison – to think just a few years ago we felt so alone in all this. Of course we had a handful of critics – people who said we were exploiting Dad, 'the son is in it for himself'. If only they knew.

If Dad didn't have music, if Dad didn't sing, he would have been in a dark place. Music is his passion – and it's the thing that keeps him going every single day. He may not have fully understood that he made an album or why people wanted photos of him, but he enjoyed every single minute of it. And that, to us, was the most important thing. The choice is either Dad sitting in a chair all day and watching daytime TV, or spending the day with his records, singing away and planning what to sing onstage. I know what I would choose.

When I wrote this book, Dad's illness was changing every day. Back then, we were in the middle of a good spell, with lots of laughs and just a handful of aggressive periods. He was incredibly caring, especially towards Mum. Of course, he was very confused, but calmer. He didn't know who I was, or Mum some days, but he knew he had a connection with us and he cared about us deeply, as we do him. To him, the real 'Simon' still lived in London. He'd often sit next to me and ask: 'Where do your mum and dad live?' I would say: 'You're my dad.' And he would reply: 'I know that. But who's your dad?' It was a pointless conversation and we'd go round and round for hours with it. But then he'd often tell me: 'Your dad must be really proud of you and how you help out me and Linda…' For me, that was worth more than all the money in the world.

Writing this book was one of the greatest gifts I've been given. I learned so much about Dad. To think that he could have quietly slipped away and I would have been none the wiser about who he was, where he came from, or how he felt about me. Like Dad, I was never brought up to value material things. 'All that matters, Sime, is that you're happy,' he would say. I may not have a designer flat in the Docklands, drive a top-of-the-range car or travel on luxury yachts, but I felt like the richest man on the planet. Who would have thought that singing along with Dad on a trip to the shops could have changed our lives in so many ways?

Through everything, my friends were a constant source of strength. I cannot count how many hours I spent going through the madness with them, sometimes in tears. They know who they are.

My mother, Linda, is the strength that has kept everything together. She is my dad's primary carer and, without her, I'm not sure what we would have done. Sometimes I wonder how she does it. But she does.

Also, I cannot end this book without acknowledging the support of the Alzheimer's Society – specifically the anonymous woman at the end of a phoneline. When it felt like life was falling apart and there was nothing left, her words picked me up and gave me the courage to continue. For that I am eternally grateful.

Finally, for anyone who's going through this: you may feel alone, you may feel like you're sinking, but you're not. You will get through it, even though, right at this moment in time, you feel like you won't. Someone once said: 'The universe gives challenges to those people it knows can overcome them.' You are one of those people. In the future you will look back at these times and realize that no matter how tough they were or how difficult you found them, they were your glory days. You coped. You blundered your way through. You made your own rules. But you got through.

So, don't give up – life isn't perfect. It isn't filtered Instagram streams or Photoshopped sunsets. Ignore that. That isn't life.

Life can be a challenge – don't be afraid. Dare to accept it.

It might not be glamorous but it's real.

And it may just take you on the greatest journey you'll ever know.

Don't Let the Good Times Pass You By

I sit beside Dad on the same sofa that Mum and Dad have had for years, trying to write. These days, the sofa has been raised up six inches by four 'elephant feet' to help Dad get up from the chair more easily – although he rarely stands up unaided anymore. Mum's in the kitchen, washing up. *The One Show* is playing on TV, just as it is every night. Dad's eyes stare off into the distance, deep in thought.

'You alright, Ted?'

'Fink so…'

I sometimes call Dad 'Ted' now. It began a few years ago, when he stopped responding to 'Dad'. It knocked me at first, when he stopped reacting to the only name I'd ever called him by. *How could he forget he was my Dad?* Instead of replying, he would join me in shouting 'Dad!' out loud and we would end up in an endless loop. Perhaps he saw me as one of his brothers. Or sisters. Misgendering happens a lot in our house these days, but rather than correcting Dad, I let it bring a smile to my face as I listen to him talk about Mum and how beautiful 'he' is. The joy in the everyday.

I'm staring down at my laptop. Eight years have passed since I sat down to write this book, and it's been a long time since I reflected on what happened when Dad first got ill. Re-reading some chapters has brought back a flood of forgotten emotions. The rage that we endured from Dad surprises me – *was it really that bad?* I guess things fade over time and we have been on a rollercoaster of a journey since then.

One thing that never fades is the pain of watching Dad change before our eyes. He now needs help with everything – feeding, washing and personal care. Some days he's connected, while on others he can be quiet, looking blank and concerned; he needs a lot of reassurance that everything's OK and that he's not alone. It's an aching reminder of how he's slipping away.

Writing this book was my therapy. My Great Reset. I was able to look at the past from older eyes, and suddenly everything fell into place. So much unexpected emotion was stirred up when I travelled down to the Black Country to research Dad's earlier life. A number of times, I'd find myself sitting in someone's front room, taking notes of their tales from the past when suddenly a wave of emotion would wash over the room. "Bloody hell, I'm starting to cry," and the tissues would come out. I then spent months in Blackburn Library, pouring everything back out into the laptop. Homeless guys and college students would become familiar faces.

'Hiya, y'alreet?' we'd parrot back the standard Blackburn greeting to each other, but thirty minutes after opening my computer, I'd find myself hiding behind the desk-divider, crying my eyes out, overcome with emotion as I poured out the stories from the past.

'You OK?'

'Yeah, I'm fine.'

But the truth was, those stories hit me hard. They reminded me of where I came from – a land I had forgotten after years of trying to fit in within the wilderness of London. *'A strange and exotic land… where the sky was always grey and the food exceptionally greasy,'* to quote Jarvis Cocker. But it's a land of love, of family, of resilience and hope – all the things that truly matter. I hadn't realised how much I had drifted from my roots until those memories came flooding back.

Reflecting on it now, I feel so incredibly proud of Hilda and Maurice, my paternal grandparents. Fourteen children! How did they do it? And every one of them turned out to be a decent human being – what an incredible legacy – I'm so proud of them all.

Writing this book also made me appreciate just how much responsibility my amazing Dad took on in his younger years as the eldest of fourteen children. He was brought up to believe in family, in looking out for each other and making sure everyone was OK. He saw those traits as fundamental to being a good person, to being a McDermott, and to being British. The idea that no one should feel left out, that we're all in this together, was something his parents (and later Butlin's) drummed into him, and he did the same to me.

I remember being a kid and seeing some louts swearing and causing trouble outside the corner shop. He marched us past them, saying, 'Ignore them ratbags, Sime. They've not been brought up British properly.' It's a comment that I used to laugh about, but now it's something I try to aspire to. I hope he would be proud.

'Do you want a biscuit, Dad?'

'A kiskit?'

'Here you go...'

I open his right hand and place a Jaffa cake in it. He gently tears it in two, giving me back a half: 'That's for you,' he says and places his piece in his mouth and downs it in one.

Sitting beside Dad on the sofa now as he taps his feet on the floor, he's like a kind, caring and happy little boy. This version of Dad is a far cry from the confused, angry man who would fly off into an uncontrollable rage at the slightest thing. It makes me feel sad to think that all that aggression arose from the immense amount of fear and frustration he was holding inside. If only we had known what he was going through at the time, perhaps we all could have dealt with it better. It pains me to think about the way I handled his aggression, and I can't help but wonder if some of my reactions provoked him further. Probably. I just wish he'd been able to tell us how he was feeling. It's a lesson I carry with me now, the importance of being honest about your feelings – both to yourself and those around you.

Recently, I gave a talk about our experiences and what we went through back then. Whenever I speak about Dad's illness now, I always tell people that if they have any worries about their own memory, they should speak to those closest to them rather than ignoring it or hoping it will go away. If Dad had opened up about his fears, we would have understood what he was going through much earlier and learned how to deal with it. As I spoke, my eyes were drawn to an old man in the front row – grey slacks, pink shirt, sensible jumper – with tears streaming down his face as he silently tried to hold it together. My heart broke for him, and I desperately hope that he was able to find the courage to open up to someone about what he was going through. Men keep a lot inside and often say nothing of their personal burdens. On the other hand, maybe I got it completely wrong, and he was crying out of boredom. I'm not Mr Showbiz, and dementia talks are not everyone's cup of tea.

***

Days and months blur together these days. Dad needs constant, round-the-clock care. Mum remains his primary carer and fortunately, we're still able to care for him at home, though I don't underestimate the commitment it takes. Without her unwavering support, I'm not sure where Dad would be. He's incredibly lucky – some people have no one. We have some great carers who come to wash and dress him in the morning and again at lunchtime, then when I finish work, I handle the evening and weekend shifts. Mum is always there though, twenty-four seven, every day of the week.

'You need to live your own life, Si – it's been eight years now. Where's the time for you in all this?' some friends say to me.

I've had countless discussions about it. I know that it comes from a place of care – but this *is* my life. What's the alternative? If we were to put Dad in a home, I know he'd be confused and lonely; we'd end up visiting every day, which would defeat the point. On top of all that, there are the huge fees that we'd have to pay. Moving him to a home would terrify Dad and depress us. I also know without doubt that, if our roles were reversed and we were suffering the same fate, he would do his best to try and keep us at home for as long as possible, and I owe it to Dad to do the same for him. It's how he raised me – that we look after each other. But there is a cost to the carer; this is real life after all. There are days when I can feel detached from my peers and start to wonder about my place in the world, though I never question whether I'm doing the right thing.

This isn't meant as a criticism of those families who have taken the difficult decision to move their loved one into a care home. Everyone's circumstances are different, and what's best for one person might not work for another. I have spoken with so many sons, daughters, wives and husbands who feel an immense sense of guilt for not being able to care for their loved one at home, but they absolutely shouldn't feel guilty – it is a brave decision, and I've never known anyone to take it lightly.

When people question my decision to stay in Blackburn and care for Dad, I have my answer ready: 'It's just a part of life that we're going through right now. It is what it is,' I say on repeat. And it is.

Luckily, I have some people in my life who do get it, and can remind me why I'm doing this when the doubts creep in. One doldrum of a day, I was sat in the pub with my dear friend Martin, Eeyore-ing to him over a pint about how I felt like I was a failure, stuck in Blackburn, going nowhere, not making a difference to anyone or anything in my life. He took a sip of his pint and simply replied, 'But you are making a bloody difference. You're making a big difference to your Dad's life. You underestimate the impact it's having on him. That's more than what some people achieve. To him, you're his hero,' he said. 'And besides – you met Joan Collins.'

Thank you, Martin: you don't know how much I needed those words that day. (I told you I'd write about you in a book.) Whenever things feel like they're getting on top of me, I think back to that pint in The Royal Oak, and I am grounded again.

Making a difference. That phrase takes me back to the time I met Iris – Dad's first love – when I was researching this book. We sat together in her front room for hours talking about what Dad was like in his younger days. She passed me a photo of them both together – the first photo I'd ever seen of Dad in his youth. I was taken aback – he looked the double of me when I was the same age.

'He was lovely,' Iris told me. 'He wasn't aggressive at all, nor a Jack-the-Lad. He never got into trouble – he was brought up very strict. Everyone knew him in Wednesbury. Anything he had, he'd always hand it over to his Mom to help with the kids. He felt it was his duty to keep the family. Honestly, that's what he thought. But I used to get so worried about him when he was older.' She sighed. 'He loved his singing – he didn't have a problem with that. It was just everything else. He was just fed up of where he was in life. All his brothers had stable jobs and settled down. He just didn't think he was making a difference.'

But Dad *did* make a difference; not only to the thousands of people who he entertained with his singing, bringing Hollywood swing to backstreet clubs, but he made a difference to me. He's my Dad, and he's been my greatest influence. As he sits here beside me today in 2024, with biscuit crumbs tumbling down his top and quite clearly very confused, I am full of pride at who he is.

'You did it, Teddy Mac! You did it!' I want to shout (and I sometimes do). If only he knew. By making just one person happy or feel less alone, he justified his entire existence.

I turn back from writing and look at Dad sitting next to me. I remember during my conversation with Iris, she told me how sensitive he was. I realise now that she was right. Dad is incredibly sensitive, which is probably why he hated seeing people alone, always making an effort to talk to them. At the time, I thought it was because he was an attention seeker – but now, looking back, I think deep down he just loved people and loved life. He didn't need bags of money or material goods. His enjoyment in life came purely from connecting with people. It was never about him, despite the glory he received. Dad was given an incredible gift – to be able to entertain and bring joy. By daring to take to the stage and allowing himself to shine, it gave others permission to do so too. And, I guess, by making the effort to connect with strangers, it made him feel somewhat less alone. It's a lesson we all could learn as we increasingly lock ourselves away behind our devices.

Ultimately, I wouldn't change caring for Dad for anything. We have our moments, of course, but I like to think it's changed me for the better and reminded me what's important in life – being close to family and caring for each other is what counts; the rest is just fluff. It's what Hilda and Maurice brought Dad up on. Whenever there is a bad day, I remind myself that I do have a choice. *Would you swap a holiday in Ibiza for what you're doing now*? I ask myself. Surprisingly, the answer is always Blackburn. Ibiza will always be there, whereas my dear Dad won't. Sometimes you just have to buckle up and enjoy the ride. It might not be glamorous, but it's real, and it matters.

***

Earlier in the evening, Mum and I are sitting at the table with Dad in between us, having our tea. I feed Dad while Mum sits next to him, having hers.

'I just wish I could go back in time,' Mum says.

'What do you mean?' I ask.

'Well,' she says, her voice faltering. Then she pulls out a tissue that has been scrunched up in her sleeve and starts dabbing her eyes.

'I mean, I wish I could just go back. I feel like I understand him a lot more now.'

'You mean, you wouldn't argue as much?'

'Well, I think that's one of the things. But all this. Everything we've learned from looking after him. I think it's completely changed how I think of him and of who he is,' she says. 'But I guess I wouldn't change anything, really, because if I did, we wouldn't all be here now.'

Of course, if we could, the one thing we would both change would be Dad having dementia. It's a cruel irony that, without his dementia, Dad and I wouldn't have reconnected in the way that we did. If he hadn't got dementia, I wouldn't have been forced to sit in a car with him trying to calm him down, driving around for hours and hours and hours. Back then, I was dealing with a breakup after a series of bad decisions. I struggle to recognise the person I was back then. I was living in a London bubble; blissfully cocooned in a drunken haze of over-priced pints and disco smoke. I was totally unprepared for real life, and none of us were prepared for Dad's illness. I felt lost, and on top of everything else, I was trying to deal with Dad's constant aggression at home. Then the universe conspired to take me back up North, squashing us into my Mum's tiny red Citroen C2. Those hours spent driving around the Tolkienesque Lancashire countryside, singing along to old big band songs with my Dad were exactly what I needed at exactly the right time. It was me who was rescued, not only my father.

A few years back, I gave a talk about the journey we had been on. Afterwards, a man approached me: 'You've had a profound spiritual experience – you just don't know it yet,' he said, and began talking to me about Jesus. I thought he was nuts and I tried to get away from him as fast as I could. But he was right.

Now, after years of reflection, I understand completely what he means. Without doubt, something was watching over us when things were at their worst – we were picked up, wrapped up and catapulted to extraordinary heights. Since then, I've lost count of how many times I've prayed to an unknown being in the sky: 'Please, God, just let us get through this.' And we do. Sometimes He does surprise you, whoever or whatever you consider 'Him' to be.

All things are possible for those who believe.

***

There's so much more I want to say about what came next after the Pride of Britain Awards. It truly was an extraordinary time for all of us. Dad's story went global, and it became the norm to have TV crews from around the world sitting in Mum and Dad's lounge. We had a ton of offers for Dad to appear on primetime shows, but I just couldn't take the risk – throughout it all, my priority was to preserve Dad's dignity. It might have made great TV to have Dad kicking off on camera or forgetting the words to a song, but at what cost? There are times that I question if I made the right decision, though – was I holding him back? Should I have taken the risk? If Dad had a good day, he would have excelled at them all.

One of the proudest moments throughout it all was seeing Dad switch on Blackburn Christmas Lights in 2016. The day before, we were sure we'd have to cancel because of Dad's confusion, but the day arrived and he was on top form, so we took the chance. I stood backstage, stifling a full-on panic attack beside a group of dancing Stormtroopers from *Britain's Got Talent* and David Platt from *Coronation Street*, while Mum and Dad chatted to the Mayor. Eventually, Dad strolled out onto the stage outside the Town Hall, announced he was an apple, tried to get me in a headlock and then went on to sing *Here in my Heart*, a cappella. There were a group of teenage lads in trackies and caps stood at the front and I fair well expected them to jeer. But instead, they stood there in silence, open-mouthed. You could hear a pin drop as Dad sang in perfect tune. When he finished, the entire crowd roared and cheered, including the lads at the front, who then started chanting, 'Teddy Mac! Teddy Mac! Teddy Mac!'

People surprise you. It was absolutely amazing.

We encouraged Dad to continue his singing as much as we could, day-to-day. The record player at home would be on constantly in the back room, but it slowly became more and more difficult for Dad to use. Eventually, Mum began taking Dad to a Singing for the Brain group organised by the Alzheimer's Society at a local church. As expected, he would end up commanding attention and would often stand at the front with Hilary, the organiser, singing away like it was *his* show. Everyone loved it and he was on top of the world.

'Come on, Mrs! You need to sing louder!' he'd shout to an old woman contorted in a wheelchair, her head slumped to one side. Those trips to the singing group were invaluable for us all. They kept Mum and Dad connected, safe in an environment where no one would judge them. But when the plate of biscuits was handed around, Dad would often refuse to pass it forward, instead stuffing as many as he could into his mouth and pockets, a flashback to his childhood, when he would take them home to share with his siblings. Of course, there were tears as Dad became increasingly confused and Mum fell more into the role of carer. Sometimes she'd be sat in the group singing away and would suddenly find herself overwhelmed by Dad's decline. The tissues would come out, followed by an understanding hug from a supportive stranger – sometimes that's all we really need to keep us going. And it did.

And it does. Over the past few years, there have been so many people who have provided countless acts of quiet, understated glory. I'd love to mention them all by name, but they know who they are – the Admiral Nurses, the social workers, the daily carers, the afternoon sitters, the church organisers, the Memory Café volunteers – all those that put in that extra something; who take the time to really listen, to pop round for a brew, to bring a smile or to lift a mood. They are the cement that keep the walls from crumbling.

Dad and I are incredibly close now. People tell me: 'I don't know what he'd do without you.' But the truth is, he's the one who's been looking after me. Having the privilege to care and spend time with him was a complete reset for my system – it's taught me a lot about life. If you have the opportunity to care for a loved one, try not to field everything out to someone else. Keep some back for yourself – you'll be surprised at the joys you will discover and the life lessons you'll receive when spoon-feeding trifle, or with elbows deep in wet wipes. These are the most precious of days, and I know that one day in the future, I will look back on them with pride.

'Tyeman, what you doing?'

'I'm writing Dad. It's a book about you…'

I used to think that Dad had forgotten who I was, but I don't think he forgot me at all – I think he just didn't recognise me – there is a difference. He knows who I am, and he knows when I'm not there, although he now calls me many different variations of my name. A few years back, in the middle of Covid, Dad stopped walking. We had no idea what started it, but I was determined that he wasn't going to just sit in a wheelchair for the rest of his life. So, each day, I would pick him up and carry him around the lounge, determined to get him walking again with baby steps as he held onto me. As I was holding him up one day, and in the midst of a babble, he suddenly looked at me directly in the eyes and shouted: 'Simon! Look at you! LOOK AT YOU! You're a man now! You're so big! You're a man!' Then he burst out laughing, grabbing my shoulders like he was the proudest man on the planet. It was an incredible experience. A second later, he went back to his confused self. It's such a baffling illness.

★★★

The cheery chorus of electronic trumpets signals the end of *The One Show*. I give up trying to write, shut the laptop and decide to add more when I get back home.

'Come on Dad. It's bedtime now.'

I stand up, facing Dad on the sofa, then bend forward and pick him up, using the same technique I use to throw forty kilo sandbags over my shoulder at the gym – one of the few things that keeps me sane these days. He feels incredibly light – *was he always this small*? The quickest way to move him to his bed in the front room is to waltz him backwards, his arms around my shoulders, mine bear-hugged around his waist.

'I've got you, I've got you, don't worry!' I shout.

It looks like a routine the Chuckle Brothers would do, but it's an easy manoeuvre and he seems to expect it now, happily "Toot-Toot-Tooting" all the way from the lounge to the front room without a care in the world, while I use all my strength not to drop him or trip over his feet.

Mum helps as I sit him on his bed. We work together to change his clothes, wash his face, smarten his hair and brush what's left of his teeth. He chats away in a babble of jabberwocky like a happy little boy – gone are the days when he would be swinging for me when we first had to do this.

'Right, Ted, I'm going to lift you up now.'

'Where we going?'

Even in his confusion, he still wants to go to the club.

'We'll have a nice sleep now and then tomorrow we'll get up and do some singing.' I sound like an old woman.

'Ohh-kayyy.'

I bend down and lift him gently into bed. Mum helps me as we layer the blankets over him. He's completely covered up, his head buried underneath the sheets, just as he's always done since he was a child. Mum picks up his old clothes and takes them into the back room to wash, leaving me and him alone.

'Right, where's my friend?' I ask.

There's no response. He's pretending to be asleep; I'm pretending to find him – this has become our nightly routine.

'Where's Ted?! Where's he gone? Dad?!'

I put my hand under the covers and ruffle his hair.

'Here he is. Here's Ted! Here's my friend!'

'What we doin?'

'It's bedtime now. I'll see you in the morning!'

'We do some singaling?'

'Yeah, we'll do it tomorrow.'

I stroke his head once more, cover him back up, pick up my bag and walk to the door.

'Tyeman?' comes a child-like voice from underneath the blankets.

'What Dad?'
There's silence.
'Dad?'
Still no response.
'Dad – what do you want?'
'Tyeman?'
'Yes Dad…'
'You're the best.'
'So are you Dad…I'll see you tomorrow.'
And I switch off the light.

Acknowledgements

This book would not have been possible without the help of the following people who gave life to the events and stories within this book.

My aunts and uncles: Chris, Joyce, Mary, Colin and Brenda, Fred and Edna, Gerry and Gill, Jane and Tony, John and Margaret, Joyce and Paul, Karen and Richard, Marilyn and Derek, Maurice and May.

Massive thanks to Ben Beards for his stories about The Starliners; Iris and Janet for sharing with openness and honesty; Barry Bennett (Baz) for his brilliant tales about the Butlin's Tour; Brian (Wardie) and Gail for Dad's Butlin's memories; the Blackburn showbiz team: Andy McKenzie, Colin Hilton, Ernie Riding and Rose Boothman for the behind-the-scenes info; Geoff, Gill and Harry for the offstage tales; Tom Lewis, Alex Van Ingen and Guy Barker – for taking a guy with dementia on a magnificent journey.

Thank you to the Alzheimer's Society for their support during the rollercoaster ride of publicity, and to the hundreds of people who have made donations or bought Dad's album through www.songaminute-man.com. The JustGiving page is still going: www.justgiving.com/songaminute

The brilliant Mary ('Write everything down!') – thank you! The superb Carly, Rachel, Marleigh (for the opportunity to refresh this story) and Lisa at HQ for making this happen.

My friends (you know who you are) for the sofas, the brews, the moans and the LOLs. For Mum, for putting up with everything life's thrown at her in the last few years and still managing to smile.

Finally, thanks to Dad, Teddy Mac. The stories he told throughout my youth formed the foundations of this book. 'You're too good-looking to be a fighter – you'll most likely be a writer' he once scrawled in my favourite book. I guess that's that ticked off then, Dad.

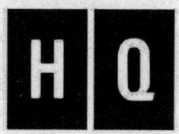

ONE PLACE. MANY STORIES

Bold, innovative and
empowering publishing.

FOLLOW US ON:

@HQStories